Mapping the
Victorian Social Body

SUNY series, Studies in the Long Nineteenth Century

Pamela K. Gilbert, editor

Mapping the Victorian Social Body

Pamela K. Gilbert

STATE UNIVERSITY OF NEW YORK PRESS

Published by
State University of New York Press, Albany

© 2004 State University of New York

For information, address State University of New York Press,
90 State Street, Suite 700, Albany, NY 12207

Production by Marilyn P. Semerad
Marketing by Jennifer Giovani

Library of Congress Cataloging-in-Publication Data

Gilbert, Pamela K.
  Mapping the Victorian social body / Pamela K. Gilbert
    p. cm. — (SUNY series, studies in the long nineteenth century)
  Includes bibliographical references and index.
  ISBN 0-7914-6025-8 (alk. paper) — ISBN 0-7914-6026-6 (pbk. : alk. paper)
    1. Medical geography—Great Britain—History—19th century—Maps. 2.
  Cartography—Great Britain—History—19th century—Maps. 3.
  Cholera—India—History—19th century—Maps. 4. AIDS (Disease)—Africa—Maps. 1. Title.
  II. Series.

G1811.E5G5 2004
614.4'0941'09034—dc21

                                                                          2003055013

10   9   8   7   6   5   4   3   2   1

CONTENTS

ILLUSTRATIONS

PREFACE

IN 1844, WHEN DICKENS'S young architect Martin Chuzzlewit visits America, he invests in Eden: "a most important place" which he knows only through a map, or, more precisely a plan. The plan shows "A flourishing city. . . . An architectural city, too! There were banks, churches, cathedrals, market-places, factories, hotels, stores, mansions, wharves; an exchange, a theatre; public buildings of all kinds, down to the office of the Eden Stinger, a daily journal; all faithfully depicted in the view before them" (*Martin Chuzzlewit* 355). Phiz's illustration shows us Martin, entranced before the great plan, as his less educated but more sensible companion Mark looks on dubiously, and the con artist selling property in Eden laughs slyly at them both. Martin buys in, of course, and shortly thereafter arrives in "Eden"—a swamp with a few "rotten and decayed" shacks in which most who have tried to build have died of fever (380). The illustration of his arrival, entitled "The Thriving City of Eden as it Appeared in Fact" pictures Martin seated before a tumbledown cabin, weeping.

Three important themes emerge in this little comedy: the idealism of the young professional intent on building the more perfect society; the contrast between the ideal society of the future and present reality expressed in terms of order and commerce versus disorder and disease; and finally, the importance of visual representation in picturing both that reality and the ideal. Here, it is the ideal which is "faithfully represented," not the reality—it is, after all, a plan, not a map. But the mapping of the ideal gives form and credibility to Eden in part because it is the goal of the young Victorian professional to civilize savagery, to turn the disease-infested swamp into the modern architectural, or planned, city. This modern city is a place of production, commerce, amusement, and above all, civility, as public buildings and a newspaper complete the references to the flourishing public sphere of Eden. Sadly, this Eden is in fact unsalvageable, but its purgatorial qualities do lead to Martin's salvation, as his selfishness and desire for easy glory in America give way to a more selfless and realistic commitment to sustained effort in Britain.

The figure of the map that appears in this vignette is an important one. As Lynda Nead points out, London's modernity was "shaped by the forces of two urban principles: mapping and movement," and the mapping had always as its goal the restoration or enhancement of that movement, usually figured as circulation (13). Sanitary mapping, such as that of sewerage, tended to figure the city as a body that could sicken (Nead 15). And the antimodern—the old, dirty slums of great cities—were figured as disease producing "Town Swamps," as George Godwin, editor of *The Builder*, put it. As Peter Stallybrass and Allon White have argued, the nineteenth-century city is organized around the binaries of filth/cleanliness and the constant fear of their transgression, or contamination, resultant from desire (136). This fear "was articulated above all through the 'body' of the city," which had to be surveyed to be controlled (Stallybrass and White 125–26). By the midcentury, this surveillance—equated with the very essence of civilization—was institutionalized in the mechanisms of sanitary inspection and had entered both literary and visual culture, the latter principally in the form of sanitary maps.

The sanitary movement responded to overcrowding and epidemic disease by emphasizing the dangers of filth. Wastes were no longer simply by-products of the life process, but animated and hostile filth that would, given the chance, attack the body itself. The body and its continence, which also modeled the boundaries of the middle-class individual self, could only be preserved through a careful policing of the abject and the closure of the boundaries of the body, through which contaminated or contaminating fluids should neither enter nor escape. By midcentury, the "lower bodily strata" of the city and its inhabitants that Stallybrass and White describe being identified with both sewage and underclass behaviors was increasingly thematized as disease and antimodernity, as health and modernity in turn came to be identified with a careful mapping and containment of the city's (and citydwellers') "guts." Sanitary mapping both documented the horrors of the modern city and provided a template for its salvation through urban planning and reform. Both Martin's optimism about the plans of Eden and his companion's skepticism refer to an increasingly complex understanding of the relationship of recalcitrant realities to these two-dimensional templates for diagnosis and improvement.

In recent years, there has been an explosion of interest in geography. Theorists of space such as David Harvey, Michel de Certeau, and Henri Lefebvre have fascinated cultural studies scholars: marxists have emphasized a return to a spatial and materialist understanding of culture; historicists, following Foucault, have insisted on the importance of geographies; and geographers, inspired by J. B. Harley, have called for a carefully theorized understanding of the historical and epistemological importance of maps. In literary studies, a new emphasis on space in narrative has emerged in numerous theoretical studies. Franco Moretti's celebrated work has carefully mapped mid-nine-teenth-century novels, seeking in their geographies new insights into the rela-tion of narrative and space. Recently, Lynda Nead has identified mapping as one of two keys to British notions of urban modernity, and sanitary mapping as a crucial use of this technology. Erin O'Connor notes of cholera, the spur to much sanitary mapping, that it "became the operative term in an entire metaphorics of bodily contamination, a figure for the fluidity of boundaries in metropolitan space" (41). Few literary and theoretical works, however, have combined these concerns, engaging maps and geographic narratives them-selves as primary cultural documents. Except for brief discussions by O'Con-nor and Nead, there has been no work examining medical maps in the light of new perspectives at all—in fact, no work that has engaged such maps as a primary topic ever, outside of highly specialized descriptive work in the his-tory of cartography.

Yet the nineteenth century was a period dominated by such mapmaking. In the late eighteenth century, as a result of imperial expansion and new tech-niques of triangulation, cartography emerged as an important—and soon dominant—mode of knowledge. With the appearance of urban epidemics and cholera in particular, medical mapping, a form of thematic cartography, became an important part of the discourses of both public medicine and urbanism. The sanitary movement attracted attention to such maps from a public larger than simply that of the medical profession, as public medicine became fundamental to governing the social body. By the mid-nineteenth century, the impact of medical maps can be seen clearly in Dickens's *Bleak House* and *Our Mutual Friend*, for example. Later social mapping and the emerging vision of London as a metropolis were shaped by early sanitary and medical maps; this foundation continued to resonate through the late-nine-teenth-century Booth maps and even in urban theory today.

This volume seeks to address the gap outlined above, at a moment when these topics are drawing particular interest. It combines attention to medical and social maps, sanitary mapping narratives, and literature to demonstrate the impact of such representations on nineteenth-century understandings of space. The social body, a concept of increasing importance in this period, in which liberal government was coming to be understood as primarily a process of understanding and managing population with the goal of a more perfect realization of that population's potential—for health, productivity, and so forth—was persistently spatialized and represented in terms of geography, especially urban geography. These knowledges were increasingly represented, then, in spatial terms, whether verbally or, as often happened, in actual maps and cartograms that both charted the condition of the population and ges-tured toward a more perfect or ideal arrangement of space. This book will be concerned with detailing the history of some of these maps in both England

and British India, along with examples of some of the other texts and discourses which depended upon or responded to them, and exploring the reorganization of social space which they both documented and contributed to. Specifically, we shall examine the development of the understanding of the social body as a concept specifically tied to an emerging vision of modern, abstract space populated by modern, structurally equivalent bodies.

The social body, as elaborated by Foucault, Poovey, and others, refers to the metaphorical description of the population as a unified and specifically corporeal whole. Although this concept had a long history in the early modern period, it took on a particular importance in the late eighteenth and early nineteenth century, as discussions of the social body coincided with a new view of the role of the state as manager of physical health and facilitator of social cohesion. With the advent of new statistical practices to canalize and measure the population, recasting it within a grid of closely related knowledge-gathering and mangement practices *(savoirs)*, the social body came to be understood increasingly as a mass of standardized and deviant bodies, making up a whole whose health was dependent on the essential equivalence of its parts. This notion of equivalent bodies was related to a notion of fundamentally equivalent subjectivities, which emerges most clearly in late eighteenth- and nineteenth-century liberalism. This equivalence is not social equality but the equivalence of an innate self, prior to culture, that is "naturally" similar across classes and that naturally manifests certain desires (for shelter, financial security, cleanliness, etc.). When the subject does not manifest those natural desires, ill health, moral, economic and political, is the result.

Poverty and vice, then, were reconfigured as less the result of a fallen nature than of the perversion of human nature through unnatural circumstances, such as living in the conditions contingent upon urban poverty. Moral health came to be seen as contingent upon, as well as coterminous with, physical health. The advent of epidemic disease in urban areas lent both focus and urgency to this understanding of the social body, as well as providing it with a vocabulary based in the notion of a physically healthy body as the basis of the modern state. The advent of modern space—gridded, uniform, and standardized—was the ideal of a government that conceived of the subjects acting in that space as structurally equivalent and behaviorally similar. Healthy subjects acting rationally would use that space in appropriate ways; in turn, the idea of a rational subject whose behaviors were statistically predictable contributed to the notion of the transparency of modern space—the ability to "know" (metaphorically and actually to *see*) the properties of spaces and subjects because of this essential similarity. Medical maps both represented the failure of the current social body to attain this transparency and indicated the steps necessary to achieve it.

The nineteenth century was the age of urban development in Britain, and perhaps no area was so compulsively mapped and narrated as London—capital city and metropole of empire. Some of the earliest attempts to theorize the peculiar nature of new urban phenomena were bound up in social and medical mapping, and a most important impetus for such mapping was epidemic disease—especially cholera, the new epidemic that became the linchpin of sanitary campaigning. This book limits its focus to spatial representations that responded to these epidemics, and their implications in relation to a larger narrative of liberal progress of which they were a part.

The book progresses in four sections, each with its own focus. The first chapter stands alone as introductory matter, situating the book's theoretical investments and providing background on material that may be unfamiliar to many readers. The second and third chapters focus on English cholera mapping, particularly of the metropolis, exploring the increasingly privileged nature of spatial representation in this period and elaborating the rise of this form of representation over the course of the period. The third section, containing two chapters, examines spatial representation in some of its cultural and narrative contexts—the reception of Snow's maps, for example, and their relation to other ways of understanding the city, and the interpenetration of sanitary mapping's spatial knowledges and the realm of fiction. The fourth, containing the last two chapters, explores the racial and spatial dichotomies of these knowledges as they were applied during the same period domestically and in British India. The parallels and divergences of medical mapping in the metropole versus the colony have much to tell about the institutional and representational history of colonial medicine in its relations to the center.

The spread of maps as tools for understanding the environment and the population paralleled a spatialization of govermental knowledges *(savoirs)* of the social body. Using the works of spatial theorists, especially of Rose and Osborne and of Lefebvre, we can understand the use of maps as a way of examining perceived and conceived social space and attempting to enforce a closer match between them. That is to say, social mapping, especially the sanitary and medical mapping with which this book shall be concerned, enabled mappers to both represent what they perceived to be before them and, by implication, an ideal to which the territory represented could hopefully be made to conform. It also enabled map readers to measure the distance between the two conditions. Thus, these spatial representations were implicated in narratives of progress; this implied relationship between a present and future state develops from one that is merely implicit in earlier, sanitarian representations, to one increasingly embedded in a historical narrative of geographic change and expert professional intervention in later, specifically medical representations. The first chapter explores these concepts. It introduces no new primary material, but provides background on the context of mapping in nineteenth-century England and its development and distribution, as well as on the disciplinary and theoretical placement of this study in the histories of medical geography and cultural studies.

Chapters 2 and 3 begin our focus on the particularities of nineteenth-century maps, tracing the specific development of sanitary and medical spatial representation in England. The first of the two surveys the earliest mappings and the reports they illustrated, their rhetorical connection of civilization with health and the mapping of that "civilized" state—or its lack—onto urban geography.[1] Initiated by the cholera pandemic of the early 1830s, medical mapping quickly became crucial to a particular vision of professionalism. Medics were increasingly able to use maps, which gave concrete form to the professional training they had received and the clinical vision with which they were endowed, to stake claims for themselves as experts in a kind of knowledge which had increasing claims to importance in the public sphere. Early medical mappers founded their claims to authority in the public sphere on their experience and education, but also on the connection of disease to vice, using a largely sanitary model of disease produced by filth. Using a rhetoric of civilization and barbarism, they laid out the identification of health with urban improvement, and both with moral progress and civilization, as well as staking the claims of medical professionals to be spokespersons for progress and civilization.

In the midcentury, the work of John Snow, the medic who advanced the theory of cholera's waterborne transmission and mapped its devastating midcentury outbreak in the heart of London, represents a significant shift as it moves toward a model based on a more modern notion of medical expertise. He bases his work less on the documentation of the visually obvious and more on a scientific understanding of details which are unavailable or inscrutable to the uninitiated—thus further consolidating the unique authority of the medical professional over the interested layman. Chapter 3 examines the important transitional moment represented by Snow's theorizing of the Broad Street epidemic, in which he famously removed the handle of the Broad Street Pump providing water from a contaminated well. This event was to have lasting significance in the representation and perception of urban space and the social body in the latter part of the century. This and the following chapter also survey the tangle of theories and responses—including but not limited to maps—offering competing visions of space and the city that related to the outbreak.

Mapmaking, obviously, did not stand separately from or replace other discursive modes of knowledge, but participated in a complex interaction with other medical and sanitary narratives, local knowledges, history, and urban myth. Snow's maps were received with such interest in part because of the high-profile nature of the epidemic's location, and that fact had a significant impact on the dissemination of medical knowledge. In chapter 4, we will trace some of the narratives already in place that shaped the reception of the Broad Street map. Contestations between local knowledges, dominant sanitary theory, and urban mythology both formed the context for one of the most important epidemiological discoveries of the period and refigured contemporary visions of the city. Moving away from a model of London as a series of separate parishes or neighborhoods, medical maps came to figure the urban environment, and London in particular, as a body—an organic whole connected by hidden mechanisms of circulation, which only the professional gaze of the medical mapper would be able to read, and therefore treat. The modern, transparent city was identified with the healthy urban body, treated surgically to remedy faults in drainage, containment, and so forth.

Medical mapping was, in the nineteenth century, increasingly related to intervention by a state that came to be seen as the proper guardian of public health. As David Harvey observes,

> In the context of the communities of money and capital, the legitimacy of the state has to rest on its ability to define a public interest over and above privatism (individualistic or familial), class struggle, and conflictual community interests. It has to provide a basic framework of institutions backed by sufficient authority to resolve conflicts, impose collective judgements, pursue collective courses of action, and defend civil society. . . . The gains provide a material basis for legitimate pride and loyalty to the local or national state. . . . The . . . practices of 'urban managerialism' are . . . fundamental to understanding the contemporary urban process. . . . The state, therefore, is not only a fulcrum for the articulation of place-bound loyalties and consciousness but also an apparatus that both internalizes and projects its own specific forms of consciousness. (*Consciousness and Urban Experience* 260)

The body and its health, deemed to be a social, and therefore not a political or economic issue, became a most important site of the state's self-legitimation in this period. Intervention was framed as fostering greater freedom of self-realization. (How, liberal Victorians asked, could a sick child benefit from education and exercise his or her free will to become a good citizen? Clearly a minimal standard of health must be fostered in order for the child to have the chance to choose to be a productive adult.) And such interventions were positioned as interventions in the environment, especially the urban locale. These interventions in turn fostered a changing conceived and lived relationship with local spaces, which included an increasing nationalist sense of self-definition through public works projects, including not only the oft-remarked monumentalizing tendencies of the Victorians, but no less crucially, though more prosaically, their drains, sewers, and housing projects. Subjectivity—national, bourgeois, imperial—could be read onto and through the environment, and articulated within a vision of progress narrated through the utopian restructuring of the built and natural environment, as is evident in the chapter 5 reading of Dickens.

Dickens's ongoing interest in sanitary matters is well known, and certainly *Bleak House*, in particular, has often been read in relation to his interest in the spread of disease. Less attention, however, has been paid to his reaction to Snow's theories and the resulting focus on the city's water supply. The quintessential Londonist, Dickens responded directly to anxieties about London's water supply and sanitary maps of Thames pollution, using current medical knowledge to create a poetics of the city which allowed for a particular kind of bildungsroman to be mapped onto London's "body." In *Our Mutual Friend*, we see both the impact of sanitary and medical mapping on Dickens's work and his skillful application of such mapping in his own narrative. The porosity of the city and its permeability by contaminated water is troped onto the porous boundaries of the improperly contained self. Dickens's midcentury liberal individualism is rendered in terms of individual characters' success or failure to contain and develop the self. The failed individual cannot contain his body, and that body is mapped onto the degenerate city's failure to manage the city's water supply.

The conception of urban space which medical mapping embodies is one susceptible of representing liberal narratives of progress and containment, as important a force in nineteenth-century novelistic narrative as in that of public health. Dickens's tale demonstrates the extent to which sanitary and medical mappers' vision of the city had been successfully absorbed. The city appears as both a single organism, vulnerable to contamination that can cross spatial and class boundaries, and as a metaphor for the project of making, or failing to make, the modern self. The novel also provides an excellent example of another narrative form's portrayal of the conceived space of medical mappers.

Sanitary mapping sought to modernize the city, to create a utopian and fully civilized metropolis in which citizens could be perfectly free to act in accordance with their desire, and their desires would always already be the right ones: that is, they would desire domesticity, cleanliness, financial security, and civility. Within that project, areas of poverty were coded as barbaric, backwards, and vicious—dark spaces to be brought into the light of the nineteenth century. Of course, as Neil Smith, among many others, has pointed out, capitalism has required noncapitalist societies as a resource to survive; modern capitalism necessitates imperialism (95). The shrinking globe is in part a result of the need to minimize the effects of distance between these two sites. In the nineteenth century, I would argue, this involved not only the remaking of colonial physical space, about which other scholars including Alfred Crosby, David Arnold, and many others have been eloquent, but also the production of a different *conceived* space which would minimize the contradictions of the simultaneous need to retain the colonial site as one of underdevelopment and the belief that capitalism would inevitably develop that site to rival the metropole. As metropolitan England envisioned itself as a modern, at least potentially utopian space, it positioned recalcitrant elements as an inner barbarism to be rooted out. The Indian colonial landscape, however, was increasingly defined through the first two-thirds of the century as permanently dark, diseased, and barbaric.

Especially in the decade following 1857, India increasingly became the other against which Britain would define itself. The modern vision of progress, related as it was to a developmental narrative of increasing metropolitan civilization and health, invoked its opposite, the unhealthy and barbaric colony. As cholera was considered a disease endemic to Bengal, we find British medics in India struggling, first to claim the authority of experience with their insular counterparts, and later to manage—or exculpate themselves from their failure to manage—the spread of disease in the territories for which they were responsible, and which came to represent the opposite of progress and civilization as they were identified with a disease which seemed to the British to be an essential characteristic of the area. In part, as I will argue in chapters 6 and 7, this was accomplished through maps which represented this conceived space of India to insular viewers. Although early mappings of cholera in India showed clear continuities with British domestic theories of disease, it began to diverge significantly by the midcentury. In these later maps, the projection of barbarism onto the other could be confirmed through the construction of both the land and the people as essentially unhealthy and insusceptible to the remediation of which metropolitan public health programs were exemplary. Cholera, an "Indian" disease emerging from the Gangitic delta which also struck hard at the urban working and underclasses at home, became a symbol not only of geographic connectedness between periphery and metropole, but of a barbarism connected with a nonutopian, heterogenous, and problematic geography.

By 1867, after the International Sanitary Conference had laid the responsibility for cholera pandemics on the British doorstep, pressure on British officials in India to modernize and sanitize leads to two clearly marked trends: one, a continuing effort to address sanitary problems in India, using similar methods to those used in Britain, and the other, to deny the current scientific knowledge of cholera in Europe as inapplicable to the disease-producing and static landscape of India. The trajectory of spatial representation in India and its differences from that of Britain is revelatory of the struggles of British medics there to cope with the differing demands and aims of the colonial sanitary project. It also reveals differing attitudes towards the spaces and people they represented, and sheds light on the ways that diverse modes of spatial representation promoted varying ways of narrating the social body.

The afterword returns to the subject of London, sketching how the vision of the metropolis as organism that emerged in the sanitary maps and was revised in Snow's work became the basis for the famous 1880s Booth poverty maps and theories of urban growth. These most famous thematic maps of the century owe much of their rhetoric to earlier sanitary and medical maps and the urban concept they made possible. In analyzing the Booth maps, we see the continuation of the theme of London as a single, vulnerable body which was so clearly developed in Dickens. By this time, however, the monstrous aspect of London-as-organism begin to outweigh the hope of the healthfully connected social body under correct medical treatment, and monstrous London comes to seem both a necessary part of the nation's economic health and naturally deleterious to its social well-being. This anatomical vision of the city, and the theories of urban growth which Booth derived from it, have continued to resonate in often surprising ways in urbanism up to the present time. The end of the section will briefly suggest some of these connections, and point toward the continuing impact of the Victorian vision on our understanding of the city more than a century later.

Even today, our Edens are often constructed as bodies resisting or succumbing to degenerative disease; even today, urban social problems are conceived as barbarism, the racial and cultural other in the heart of modernity. Perhaps especially today, we inherit an intensified, evolved version of both young Martin's idealism and his author's distrust. We are seduced by the abstract logic of the two-dimensional plan and see the real landscape, with its human and geographic messiness, as an annoyingly recalcitrant weakness in the otherwise clean and modern city. The planned city seems to promise freedom, commerce, prosperity, unproblematic connection. Our simultaneous distrust of urban planning, however, no longer turns so much on the understanding of the natural environment as hostile as on a distrust of the built environment. We join the late-nineteenth-century urbanist in our suspicion that the city is not only disease producing, but damaging to our freedom and individuality. Homogenous spaces seem designed to promote homogenous subjectivities. The differences that survive sometimes seemingly serve only to encode classed and raced hierarchies. Neither these hopes nor fears are wholly unfounded. In clarifying the history of some of these representations, however, we may come to a useful understanding of the political and historical entailments that affect their explanatory value in the present day.

ACKNOWLEDGMENTS

As is usual with any project, I owe thanks to too many people to count. Institutions first: I must mention the generous assistance and friendly atmosphere of the Wellcome Institute for the History of Medicine, and especially Sally Bragg, who makes it all function smoothly. Thanks too to the Wellcome Library, London. The ever-reliable British Library, where I have had many happy hours, has made this book possible. Finally, the Public Records Office, the London Guildhall, the archivists at St. Bart's and the East London Hospital, and the interlibrary loan staff at the University of Florida all contributed to this project, as did material support from the University of Florida and the National Endowment for the Humanities.

Of my colleagues, all of whom are important sources of stimulation and support, I would like to especially thank the other Victorianists at the University of Florida: Julian Wolfreys, Chris Snodgrass, and Alistair Duckworth. My other colleagues and friends Susan Hegeman, Phil Wegner, Maude Hines, Nancy Reisman, Stephanie Smith, John Murchek, Sid Dobrin, Kim Emery, Terry Harpold, Roger Beebe, Apollo Amoko, Leah Rosenberg, Pat Craddock, Martha Bryant, Maureen Turim, and Brandon Kershner have given me invaluable intellectual, social, and emotional nourishment. Special thanks to Kenneth Kidd, who read and commented on an early stage of the manuscript, and for his unfailing enthusiasm and sense of fun, and to Tace Hedrick whose friendship and conversation sustain me. Special thanks also to the Chair of the Department of English, John Leavey, whose support has been important to this project. Of colleagues outside the University of Florida, I must thank Michael Levenson, who introduced me to London and sparked my interest in urbanism. Elizabeth Langland, although now on the other side of the continent, has continued to be a terrific colleague and mentor, as has Jim Kincaid. Of many correspondents, Talia Shaffer has been a particularly wonderful interlocutor, as have Tim Alborn, Lesley Hall, Steve Sturdy, Ryan Johnson, Susan Zieger, Yopie Prins, David Wayne Thomas, Martha Vicinus, and many others whose comments at conferences or over e-mail have been crucial to my thinking about the larger cholera project. I am particularly grateful to Mark Harrison for his comments on chapters 6 and 7, as well as his general intellectual generosity. Many graduate students have contributed to my thinking and have helped make my intellectual environment a productive one, and I'd like to thank them all, but must single out Meg Norcia, Michelle Sipe, and Heather Milton, and especially Jung Hwa Lee, whose editing assistance was invaluable. This work or work related to it has been presented at a number of conferences and working groups, where many scholars have influenced my thinking. These include the MLA, various Society for the Social History of Medicine and Wellcome conferences, the Victorians' Institute, the Workshop on Framing and Imagining Disease, the nineteenth-century group at the University of California, Berkeley and the Nineteenth-Century Studies Group at the University of Michigan.

Clare Ford Wille and Peter Shahbenderian, Londonists extraordinaires, have shared their home and their lives with me, put me on the right trains, loaned me umbrellas, and supported this and the larger cholera project unreservedly for the seemingly endless series of summer research visits it has taken to see it completed. Long phone conversations with family and friends Angela Geitner, Meryl Strichartz, and Nicolet de Rose took me over the rough spots and put things in perspective. And finally, I must thank Gustavo Verdesio, for knowing when to laugh with me, when to laugh at me, when not to laugh at all—and for many other things and much more than I can easily say.

Portions of chapters 2 and 3 and of the Afterword have appeared in "Mapping the Social Body of Nineteenth Century London," in *Imagined Londons,* edited by Pamela K. Gilbert, State University of New York Press, 2002. Part of chapter 4 was published as "'Scarcely To Be Described': Urban Extremes as Real Spaces and Mythic Places in the London Cholera Epidemic of 1854," *Nineteenth Century Studies* 14 (2000): 149–72. Material from chapter 5 appears in "Islands in a Filthy Stream: Medical Mapping, The Thames, and the Body in *Our Mutual Friend,*" *Filth,* edited by William Cohen and Ryan Johnson, University of Minnesota Press, copyright 2004 by the Regents of the University of Minnesota. Finally, materials from chapters 6 and 7 are forthcoming in "Mapping Colonial Disease: Victorian Medical Cartography in British India," in *Framing and Imagining Disease,* edited by George Rousseau, Palgrave, August 2003. Thanks again to the Wellcome Library, London, for permission to reprint specific images identified in the List of Illustrations.

PART I

Introductory

1

Mapping and Social Space
in Nineteenth-Century England

> For a perfect system of hygiene we must combine the knowledge of
> the physician, the schoolmaster and the priest, and must train the
> body, the intellect and the moral soul in a perfect and balanced order.
> —Edmund Parkes, *Practical Hygiene*

NINETEENTH-CENTURY ENGLAND saw a growing concern with what came
to be defined as social problems—poverty, crime, and what would finally be
termed "public health" issues. Much of this has been correctly attributed to
urbanization and industrialization, and the urban is certainly central in conceptions of the social body in this period, particularly London. More recently,
however, we are coming to understand the role of modern liberalism and the
state in recreating problems seen at the beginning of the century as endemic
to capitalist—or indeed any—society as problems in the development of the
citizen. These problems then could be understood not only as susceptible to
treatment but demanding it for the health of the social body.

In the Victorian period, medicine evolved fairly rapidly from a loose
assortment of ill-defined practices and practitioners identified with the private
sphere into an elite profession with increasing status in the public arena. Further, science itself became an important part of national identity, as Britain saw
itself as a scientific nation, and the Empire consciously styled itself as a ruler
through archival knowledge.[1] As Foucault has argued, the move toward modern liberal government is marked by "governmentality"—the development of
bodies of knowledge which are also practices, particularly in regard to biopoli-
tics (the management of populations) through public health, the census, and

the like. These knowledges, which were also practices, enabled governments both to know about the movements and living habits of their subjects and to mobilize consent among those subjects to governmental aims, rather than relying on brute power. The professionals who designed, managed, and were the instruments of this process of what Foucault would call "governmentality" authorized themselves with claims to be speakers for the nation, and therapeutic managers of the nation's social body. Medics and sanitarians became central to that process as social ills were displaced from the political sphere, medicalized, and reinscribed within the purview of public medicine. Public health—especially in relationship to epidemic disease and sanitary issues—has a privileged role in the discourses of the social body.

Public health emerged in this period as part of the tendency toward governmentalization; the opportunity arose in response to (particularly urban) epidemics, and cholera has generally been accorded the role of prime actor in this drama. It is important to remember that the cholera itself did not cause the public health movement—had the conditions not been right for acceptance, however grudging, of public health as the business of government, and had the beginnings of statistical knowledge not made public health as a knowledge project feasible, cholera alone would have done little. But the conditions were right, and the dramatic eruption of an alien and frightening epidemic during conditions of reform agitation provided unique practical and narrative opportunities, despite the fact that cholera was hardly as important a threat as the routine depredations of diseases already endemic to the Isles. Medics used the public attention elicited by these events to create a public platform for the profession; they mobilized discourses of nation and the social to add force to their position, and in so doing, contributed to the formation of those discourses themselves. For these reasons, public health and the cholera epidemics provide an especially fruitful source of stories about the social body. The body becomes both the sign and the metaphor of the nation. Individual bodies and their ills, as representatives of classes and populations, become indices of the condition of that less tangible entity, the social body. The social itself, in both its physical and moral manifestations, comes to be understood as a medicalized physical entity which can be fixed, observed, and dissected both through the individual bodies of its subjects and in toto (or en masse) in the form of statistics. Over time, the social body comes to be read geographically, as identical with its geographic location and built environment; public intervention in the one is both effected by and reduced to a physical, environmental intervention.

The social body was a concept increasingly associated with spatial forms of knowledge, especially geographic distributions—of mortality rates, educational level, population concentration, and so forth. This knowledge was gathered as information, but used in turn to form policy. Public health advocates saw their role not merely as improving the physical health of individuals, but as forming the moral character—closely tied to physical health and cleanliness—which in turn would produce the ideal modern citizen. Nikolas Rose, among others, has argued that the nineteenth-century understanding of the social is fundamentally both spatial and politicized (104–105). Spaces were identified with their own protocols and good citizenship was aligned with a form of self-governance which involved adhering to those protocols. For example, "Recreation was also to be spatially organized—no longer in the rowdy and transgressive hurly-burly of the market, the fair, and the baiting of bears—but in new moral habitats—public parks, municipal swimming pools. . . . [T]he space of the town became intelligible in new ways, in the spatial imagination produced by all those who thought that in order to govern relations between people more effectively one had first to inscribe them" (Rose 105). Certainly this point has been made by others as well (Poovey, *Making a Social Body*, Procacci, and so on).

Rose, unlike Procacci, chooses to emphasize the new freedoms which liberal government and its ideologies held as goals for the modern individual, whereas other theorists have tended to emphasize the restrictions posed by the panoptic penetration of subjectivity which such freedom demanded. Both of these positions have merit, of course. But both agree that such use of space as the medium of social surveillance and discipline required a reorganization of space which most scholars, following the marxian thread of Harvey and Lefebvre, have termed "abstraction." This argument holds that capitalism demanded an increasing abstraction so that unique spaces (and, implicitly, subjectivities) could be refigured in terms of structural equality and interchangeablility. Such representations, as Foucauldians have pointed out, stressed transparency and visibility. These ideal abstract spaces confronted the reality of the nineteenth-century city—opaque, heterogenous, illegible. A practice that depended on the structural equality of individuals and the natural similarity of their desires faced a heterogenous population whose natural desires seemed to have been deformed by circumstances. A vision which stressed light, openness, and circulation faced a built environment of crowded courts and cul-de-sacs.

Thomas Osborne and Nikolas Rose have provocatively defined the nineteenth-century liberal ideal of the urban space as that of "virtuous immanence"—that is to say, the city was to provide a space in which citizens exercised their freedom to govern themselves, a crucible in which competing ideals and desires would lead, naturally, to a kind of ideal state emerging from the urban fabric itself. However, they also stress, the freedom provided by the city also led to another, less socially desirable form of immanence—the "vice, rebellion, insubordination" of those whose "sociability" was imperfect (*Governing Cities* 3). Although I suspect Osborne and Rose ascribe too much sense of the city's initial legibility or rationality to nineteenth-century urbanists whose own views seem to be more along the lines that London, like Topsy, just grew (and not in any rational or even particularly viable manner), it is certainly true that early social and medical mapping of the city was aligned with efforts to understand the relationship of undesirable "forms of freedom" and the urban environment. I would argue, however, that it is not until the midcentury that Victorian urbanists began working with a fully developed sense of the city as a whole, even as an organism with its own rhythms and cycles. Mapping had a large part in that process of understanding, as it did in its next step: planning, the creation of ideal maps used to remake the city into a structure more consonant with the planner's goals. As Rose and Osborne suggest, these "diagrams" tried to make "urban existence both more like and less like a city—more in that the immanent virtues of the civic are intensified, less because the immanent dangers of the city are pacified" (*Governing Cities* 3). Their emphasis on the utopian elements of this vision are an important intervention in the predominant scholarly tendency to see such work as purely designed to suppress the freedom of the underclasses.

However, it is also important to remember that such limitations were often the undeniable result of these projects. Most of the major redevelopment projects of the nineteenth century—the Oxford Street extension known as the New Cut and abolition of the Rookery in St. Giles, for example, which drove thousands of slum dwellers out of their homes (and into even worse slums nearby)—were motivated by and argued for in terms of the social body and its health. Moral and physical problems were closely aligned and increasingly conceived in terms of interventions in the built and natural environments. Key to these developments was a naturalistic vision of the role of the social. It was largely believed that what were defined as appropriate (bourgeois) social values were innate, natural. However, the bad urban environment could deform these natural traits just as the urban environment could foster them; dirty slums gave children an acquired and unnatural taste for dirt and darkness which led inevitably to vice and disease. Rose and Osborne suggest that the nineteenth-century city was seen as an ideal laboratory of government, and that the "government of this space had to be concerned above all with the security of these natural processes of society" developing in this specifically urban environment (*Governing Cities* 7).

This understanding of Victorians' views, though, should be tempered with an appreciation for the nineteenth-century distrust of the city: its nostalgia for the rural, the upper-middle-class flight to villas outside of London, and the still-strong belief that its ruling classes should be based in large landholdings outside the city. In London, at least, the sense of the city's "immanence"—its organic ability to foster a life defined by freedom and access to goods and services which fostered a liberal notion of (self-)government—was insistently counterpoised against its long-standing image as degenerate and leading to poor self-fashioning practices. As Rose and Osborne themselves point out, the extensive literature of medical topography which emerges in the 1830s and after implies a relation between the urban and illness, and the task of urban government becomes in large part to promote health and to govern "the spatial relation between citizen and habitat" (*Governing Cities* 9). Still, Rose and Osborne tend to see the pathologizing of the urban as something that takes place principally at the end of the century with degeneration theory and "the novel question of overcrowding" in homes, which they believed emerged in the 1880s (*Governing Cities* 13). In fact, it emerges quite a bit earlier and is in full flower in the 1850s. In short, in tracing the origin of the nineteenth-century city to the city-states of ancient Greece, Rose and Osborne have perhaps somewhat oversimplified the relationship between urban and rural, metropole and nation in nineteenth-century England. However, this makes no difference to the core implication of their very fine analysis, which is that the freedom and concentration of population of the city were both perceived as the quintessential characteristics of the utopian urban impulse—the city's modernity and the multiplication of what Rose and Osborne call possibilities for sociability—and of its destructive and unhealthful nature.

Early to midcentury urban planning sought to meliorate or fine-tune what was already extant in the city, at first in despair of any larger possibilities, and later with more sense of the utopian possibility of an inclusively planned space. The urban was inextricably identified with a massed and dangerous, yet necessary social body which must be observed and medically optimized; this medicalized urban population became the sign and goal of modernity and progress on which the British sense of imperial entitlement depended. Sanitary surveys and mapping, later to become more formally medical mapping (that is, a mapping dependent upon specifically professional forms of expertise) became an important part of this envisioning and disciplining of the urban (and national) social body. Mapmaking sought to make visible what was invisible, to simplify spatial information by subjecting it to the abstracting process of mapmaking. This process eliminated extraneous information and reduced complex, obscure spaces to clearly understandable lines and symbols subject to a consistent series of measurements. Initially, much of such mapmaking simply illustrated a set of data and, sometimes, an explicit argument about its meaning. Over the course of the period, it came to be used both diagnostically—to show what was lacking—and more and more unequivocally in planning—to gesture toward a utopian realization of the liberal narrative of progress. In doing so, it gestured towards two levels of social space simultaneously, what Henri Lefebvre, in *The Production of Space*, has called "perceived" and "conceived" space.

Most theorists of space posit two types of space superimposed on or coexisting with each other: physical space and social space (what Neil Smith, in *Uneven Development,* calls relative space). Physical space encompasses both the natural or "given" and the built environment, and of course, as Smith points out, nature is itself produced, both ideologically and physically, through human interaction with the land, and through various scientific practices which seek to measure it.[2] In social space, Lefebvre identifies a threefold split: perceived, conceived and lived social space, among which there is a complex interaction. Perceived space is space as we practically understand it and act on it; conceived space is space as we represent it, through various scientific and other knowledges; and lived space is that which we actually experience from moment to moment, mediated through culture, psychology, and so forth (*Production* 36–42). In this layered space, notes Lefebvre, exist multiple contradictions generated by the dialectic practices of space by human beings operating simultaneously in all of these levels.

In this book, I shall be principally concerned with the conceived space of medical mapping but, as Lefebvre suggests, it is impossible to deal with this level of social space without the intrusion of lived and perceived space. Thus, although our primary concerns are with the ideologies of knowledge production, we shall also see how the lived experiences and perceptions of those who inhabited these various spaces interacted with the conceptions of mappers (especially in chapter 4, treating the relationship of St. Giles and St. James's parishes). Conceived space in this period, was, according to Lefebvre, increasingly abstract, and is characterized by Euclidean rationality (which dictates that all heterogenous spaces are reducible to certain absolute and homogenous terms), a privileging of visual ways of knowing which deemphasizes other sensoria, and what he calls the "phallic formant," a use of altitude and the "god's eye view" to enforce a sterilizing abstraction which, he believes, is itself a form of brutality (*Production* 285–91). The focus on abstraction, however, brings us back to Rose and Osborne's view that to some degree, this abstraction is also the basis for liberalism, with its apparent cherishing of the ideals of freedom and autonomy. A certain amount of homogeneity in the desires and practices of individuals are, as we have said, theorized as necessary for the personal freedom that underpins liberalism. Perhaps the difference between the modern liberal state and less desirable forms of modern government (fascism, for example) depends in part on the fine balance between the mobilization of consent and direct coercion—perhaps, Rose and Osborne's work suggests, there is even a relation between the more perfect realization of a certain "abstraction," a consequent lack of need for coercion, and the perceived accrual of increased freedom.

An important—perhaps the most important—project for envisioning the social body emerged through what would later be called public health.

Spurred by cholera epidemics, and building on the evaluation of individuals' productive capacity in terms of health and longevity that political economy had naturalized, sanitarians and medics began to conceive the population as an entity subject to certain common influences on mortality and morbidity. As physical and moral well-being were interwoven, these arguments encompassed the causes of not only physical illness, but of vice. Nineteenth-century sanitary and medical mapping concerned themselves with identifying and eliminating pockets of disorder, overpopulation, and working-class behaviors coded as vice and as disease in order to bring the city under a grid of manageability. To do that, mappers first had to conceive an ideal mental map of any given space, a map based on attributes conceived as universally desirable. In this way, the specificity of some spaces came to be seen as pathological; what would be desirable would be conformity to universal standards of cleanliness, drainage, population concentration, and so forth which were common to and interchangeable within all spaces.

The ability to represent any lived environment two dimensionally, with reference to the presence or lack of these universal desiderata—that is, in a sanitary map—was basic to the insertion of that space into a narrative of social progress and urban wholeness which would in turn be based on the conversion of that space into one matching the ideal. Every step toward totalizing that vision was, in the eyes of both sanitarians and medics, a step toward the "virtuous immanence" Rose and Osborne cite—or, if one prefers, toward the totalizing abstraction decried by Lefebvre. For the conversion of spaces did not only imply a physical change to the built environment, but a moral and social change to the population mapped onto and held by it. Part of that process was bringing the general population's *perception* of space into closer alignment with medics' *conception* of space—that is, sanitary education sought to make the general population view as desirable the light, dryness, cleanliness, and openness of circulation that sanitary mappers viewed as desirable.

Yet as such mapping, and particularly mapping of disease, became more complex and more clearly based on specialized medical knowledge in the 1850s, it also came to stand in for the inability of the general public to see that which only a trained professional could make clear. In other words, mapping's increasingly specialized concerns stood as an argument for the yielding of public authority over urban improvement to medics and engineers. Increasingly, such mapping came to be seen not simply as either illustrative or persuasive, but as diagnostic, a way of seeing which, though objective, would itself yield knowledge, rather than simply representing it. Over the course of the century, as attention shifted from sick populations to sick geographies which came to symbolize both the environment and the population mapped onto it, these geographies—especially urban ones—were conceived increasingly as large bodies themselves. By midcentury, circulation, particularly of water and sewage, was perceived as systems unifying dispersed areas and populations into one organic whole which could be anatomized, mapped, and treated "surgically"—through engineering intervention and public works projects which would alter those hidden circulatory mechanisms—to become healthy, modern, rational, and transparent.

MAPPING IN ENGLAND

In order to situate the present study, I would like to pause here for a background discussion of mapmaking in the period, how it progressed, and why it became particularly prominent in the public imaginary at this time. (Those readers not particularly interested in the history of mapping and its techniques may want to skip ahead to the next chapter.) After all, the concept of population as an aggregate had been around for some decades; why do certain kinds of spatial representations emerge at this time? Britain, like other European powers, had long been a mapmaking culture. During the Enlightenment, maps came to embody the power of the objective, scientific gaze to construct—or reflect—an accurate description of the geographic environment. Imperialism gave new force to mapmaking as a science, as exactness of measurement and topographic descriptions came to have new importance both for military actions and public works. The development of techniques of triangulation in the eighteenth century enabled cartographers to construct measurements with impressive precision. Matthew Edney, speaking of the survey maps of India, remarks that triangulation "implicitly created a natural cartographic space to be filled with natural symbols: consistency of representation would derive automatically from consistency in observation and measurement . . . the perfect geographic panopticon . . . because its geography would be the same as the world's. . . . [I]t promised such an improvement that the archive became definitive" (337).

Both within and outside Britain, mapmaking flourished with an enthusiasm that at one point led the Ordnance Survey to attempt mapping of urban areas in Britain at a scale of ten foot to the mile! (This ambition was later significantly reduced to forty inches to the mile.) Meanwhile, new developments in lithography enabled maps to be created and disseminated more cheaply than ever before. By the early to mid-nineteenth century, maps were everywhere—in schoolrooms, as frontispieces to books, in journals and so forth. By the time railways were in common use for business and personal travel, thus shrinking the world, maps were a type of spatial representation to which many Britons had some recourse in envisioning their environment.

Human beings use many cognitive strategies for representing and practicing (acting in) space. The most important ones for our daily lives seem to be experiental, having to do with the way we interact with objects, spaces, and places (spaces invested with and constructed by meanings)[3] on a regular basis in what social geographers call space/time—that is, since our interactions with space have a chronological element, our perceptions of space differ according to time—of day, of year, of the lifecourse. Golledge notes that individuals' "place recognition may often be *descriptively rich* but *spatially inaccurate*," (his emphases, 412). Supplementary to these mental representations, and becoming increasingly important in proportion to our lack of direct personal experience and to the size of the area in question, are shared external representations—maps of various kinds—which individuals internalize in differing ways.[4]

Widely shared maps of this type, then, perform an important function in defining communities—not only spatial communities, but interpretive and identity-based communities. Although the role of maps in promoting nationalism has been rather extensively discussed, it is good to bear in mind that simple access to urban maps construct—and situate—the map user as an urban dweller in ways very different than experiental cognitive mapping might dictate. For example, a person whose work and home life were based in Islington in 1830 and who had either no resources or no compelling reasons to do much travel might have a very clear, detailed, spatially and chronologically accurate sense of Islington and surrounding areas, but only a hazy sense of the geography of Westminster and very little sense of the relative proportions and locations of various localities in East London. Awareness of a formal map of London might provide such a reader with a quite different sense of location vis-à-vis the city as a whole than the reader had previously entertained. To what extent this would have any cognitive impact on spatial understanding would depend on personal factors as well as on any experiental reason for internalizing the information. Individuals who had no interest in say, Whitechapel, might quickly forget its position relative to their own; others, perhaps having a relative who had lived there, might retain it to the exclusion of any information about surrounding areas. The thematic maps of the nineteenth century constructed space—and place, as defined by particular labels (St. James's, London, and so forth)—in ways that were meaningful to those who constructed the maps.[5] Often, this meant defining place by parish boundary. We should remember, though, in reading these maps, that such constructions often had little to do with the place definitions of those who lived in those spaces. In fact, such maps may well have served to redefine place for readers whose previous sense of boundaries may have been fluid and hazy (as Golledge shows such boundaries often are) until an authoritative representation served to fix them.

Such maps provided to those who did use them a way in which to cognitively organize their world, enabling viewers to situate themselves within various totalities—the world, Britain, a city, a parish, perhaps a neighbor-hood. Maps were widely available by the mid-nineteenth century, spreading quickly throughout European culture, even turning up in ladies' needlework patterns. A standard subject in girls' and boys' schools, sampler maps, along with multiplication tables and alphabets, were popular assignments as early as the 1790s (Tyner 3). Adult women worked decorative needlework maps as wall hangings and fireplace screens, and embroidered globes enjoyed a vogue (Tyner 6).[6]

Additionally, mapmaking was widely taught; manuals for both children and teachers sold well in the late 1840s and 1850s onward, and several were published for the use of professionals as well. Alfonzo Gardiner's *How to Draw a Map* (1879) sold for 1 shilling and was directed at pupil-teachers. William Hughes's *A Manual of Mathematical Geography Comprehending an Inquiry into the Construction of Maps with Rules for the Formation of Map-projections* (1852) sold for 3s 6d, and was used by students in schools and colleges. Inset adver-tisements in the second edition of this book offer a number of books and maps for primary school children, often to be drawn on or colored in; the maps are offered at 1–2d each. Hughes observes to his teenaged audience,

> The use of maps in illustration of different subjects is almost infinitely var-ied . . . and the frequency with which they are employed in the present day for *special* (instead of merely general) purposes . . . [is] evidence of a more extended appreciation of their true utility. . . . [M]aps . . . exhibit the . . . *localised* details of almost every phenomenon in social life. (133)

Interestingly, despite the emphasis on objectivity, students were as often taught, at least initially, to think of the maps as aesthetic objects rather than exact reproductions of the terrain, suggesting that the Victorian understand-ing of realism in cartography may have been different from ours. Gardiner's manual for map drawing for teachers urged accuracy in the broad issues but emphasized aesthetics too: under "coast Line" he suggests, "[D]o not make it too *fine*, nor too *stiff*, but rather 'wavy,' so as to indicate small indentations" and again under "Rivers and Lakes," "Always begin the source of a river with a *fine line*, making it wavy, and, as it reaches the coast, increasing in thickness. Take especial care that the rivers do not look like 'wires,'" indicating that often fine detailing on a map may be more suggestive of the genre than the actual feature it represents (4). Detailed land use maps and geological maps of Britain became available from 1800 to 1815 (Thrower, *Maps and Man* 84–85). Additionally, several geographic societies founded in the nineteenth century published many maps; new printing techniques allowed them to print them in their journals and proceedings (Thrower, *Maps and Civilization* 154).[7] By the 1850s and 1860s, Britons saw the very wide and cheap dissemination of maps in educational material, travel guides, and other such literature.[8]

London, as a world center of economic and shipping activity, as the metropole of a growing empire and capital of Britain, naturally drew much attention from cartographers, and perhaps no community provided more of a consumership for such representations than Londoners themselves. Since the beginnings of its accelerated expansion in the late eighteenth century, London had become increasingly large and various, and Londoners themselves were fascinated with the "Mysteries" of their own city. Not only did maps and guidebooks strive to give an overview of the city, but narrative mappings attempted to create an understanding of not only its physical geography, but its social structure as well, along with its various languages and other signifying practices. To this end, Londoners attended theatre productions staged in elaborate re-creations of specific London neighborhoods and landmarks, consumed dictionaries of slang and "flash" patter designed to initiate them into the mysteries of lower- and underclass communities, enthusiastically read ethnographies like Mayhew's *London Labour and the London Poor,* and entertained themselves with publications ranging from *Tom and Jerry* to the younger Charles Dickens's *Dictionary of London.*[9] London became the clearest spatial representation of Englishness, and medical mapping of London became a proportionately important mode of representing the health of the social body more generally.

The increasing visibility of maps, along with cheaper modes of production and dissemination, encouraged broader and more experimental uses of maps for specific purposes. The period from 1830 to 1855 has been termed the "golden age" of thematic mapping (Robinson, "The 1834 Maps" 440)—the use of maps to illustrate a specific dataset or argument, usually having to do with human action in space.[10] Lithography, especially the autographic technique, made printing maps cheaper and easier.[11] Most symbols and techniques in thematic cartography were in use by the 1830s and practically all in use today were in use by the 1860s (Robinson, *Early Thematic Mapping* 186). The first two were in use before the century began. Dots of variable value were used as early as 1830. Choropleth mapping, that is, dividing a terrain into blocks which are flatly shaded according to the statistical value of the region defined by the boundaries (for example, a given parish might be given a particular shade according to how far above the average the birth rate was for that parish) was first used in France in 1826. The more sophisticated isopleth method—a way of using isolines like those found on contour maps to represent statistical data—appears to have been first used in Denmark around 1854. Robinson identifies five main techniques: writing statistics on the map, dots of uniform value, dots of variable value, choropleth, and isopleth (Robinson, *Early Thematic Mapping* 110–11). The first four techniques, then, were already in common use for medical mapping by the 1830s.[12]

The most typical use of thematic mapping before this period was for military/colonial purposes, although some population, linguistic, and even medical maps were created before this time. But most cartographic historians agree that thematic cartography generally, and especially medical cartography, began in the early nineteenth century, getting a boost from outbreaks of yellow fever in the United States and becoming fully established during the cholera pandemic of the early 1830s. Cholera is generally seen as the epidemic which established medical mapping as a standard technique in Europe and the Americas and certainly in Britain (E. W. Gilbert 173; Jarcho, "Contributions" 133; Stevenson 228), and these will be the maps with which this book will be principally concerned.

Thematic mapping of this sort is essentially a statistical argument presented visually, and so was a result of the development of statistics as an important area of knowledge. However, it also came into being as a result of the spatialized understanding of social problems in this period. Before the significant use of such maps (which mapped not only disease, but also poverty, crime, religious practice, and educational access as the most common measures), written accounts already tended to describe the conditions of populations spatially, street by street and sometimes house by house.[13] In other words, social problems were already understood with reference to location, to the built and natural environment, and to proximity to areas already deemed problematic. As Stevenson observes, such detailed spatial descriptions cried out for visual representation (240). Thematic maps were created and displayed at the Great Exhibition of 1851, and by the late 1850s, if not earlier, cholera mortality maps were printed to be displayed in the registration districts.[14] These descriptions are clearly ancestors of the both comprehensive and highly localized Booth maps of the 1890s. Thematic maps allowed readers to simultaneously situate themselves in a totality of human activity or experience and a spatial totality which was connected to, and helped define, that human community. Medical maps located human beings in a community of bodies linked by common vulnerability to disease.

Medical maps, presumably, would not have been as widely consumed as, say, the Society for the Diffusion of Useful Knowledge (SDUK) maps; however, the epigraph to this chapter, taken from a sermon published in pamphlet form, implies that this minister's audience (largely middle to upper class), at least, was expected by the orator to be familiar with sanitary maps:

> Cleanliness . . . and an early application of medicine and medical skill . . . were supposed to be specifics against the contagion. . . . But pushing that truth too far, men began to map out the geographical boundaries of the malady. . . . Then the selfishness of our nature, leaving the poor in their disease or in their danger to pay the penalty of their localities, was heard to congratulate itself on the comparative safety of its better situations. (Rev. Henry Venn Elliott 9–11)

Clearly the minister speaks of both the mapping and readers' reactions as topics of common knowledge by 1855, well outside of medical circles. He also recognizes—and calls upon his auditors to recognize—the classed nature of such mapping, its social and policy investments, and deleterious effects upon the disenfranchised. This sermon implies that both familiarity with such maps and rather sophisticated mapreading practices—such as use of maps to predict one's own vulnerability to disease—were fairly widespread.

READING SANITARY MAPS

Although, clearly, overall map use was quite widespread in the middle- to upper-class population, I have found no evidence that sanitary maps were very widely perused specifically by the literate working classes. Although there was much didactic literature for the poor on sanitary living, and much educational literature with maps, the two strands seem not to have combined. Didactic literature like *Through Tumult and Pestilence,* a novel about cholera in a village, written by Emily Lawson and published by the SDUK, expects a certain familiarity among its audience with medical topography narratives. It describes the village in terms of fever-producing, low-lying areas near stagnant ditches, salubrious areas that are high and airy, and so forth, but that does not necessarily mean such readers were thought to have seen cartographic representations. And such maps were not widely reproduced in the middle-class quarterlies, even once the technology existed to do so.

Who, then, did read them? Those within the medical community who either worked with sanitary agencies or were interested in epidemiology certainly both constructed and perused these maps. Journal articles only occasionally mention maps, but when they do, they assume familiarity or at least access. In an 1849 issue of the *London Medical Gazette,* there was reprinted the first of Dr. W. F. Chambers's 1832 *Three Lectures to Students at St. George's Hospital,* which seems to have been conducted originally with the aid of maps from government reports on the cholera in India. The text assumes that Dr. Chambers's listeners have access to these maps, as he offhandedly concludes a discussion of the directions of spread of the disease with the comment, "A reference to any of the maps will show the distribution of those routes" (Chambers 293). The maps produced by the General Registrar's Office were certainly seen by law and policy makers and those social activists interested in such questions, and at least some were directed to be displayed in the registration districts. Local sanitary maps of the type used in the parish level reports on the cholera epidemics to the central authorities were very likely usually seen by the parish boards and anyone who came to their meetings. This means that a substantial minority of the elite rate-paying male population would have seen such maps—if not a disease map specifically, at least a "sanitary condition" map. These maps were also used and referred to by other report makers and by researchers like Snow. As we shall see below, popular interest in the position of the Lord Craven pest field during the St. James epidemic suggest that at least in this parish, quite a few people chose to view the map. Still, sanitary and medical maps were probably far more familiar to middle-class readers than to workers.

For those who did read sanitary maps, and who agreed with the basic assumptions which they were created to illustrate, to read such a map involved a comparison of the perceived space the map displayed (and perhaps one's own lived experience of it) to the conceived space on which the map was implicitly based. In turn, to read the map sympathetically involved the absorption of an ideal of space that was transparent to representation (such transparency itself standing in perhaps for dryness, or a certain threshold of population density past which the map would begin to darken, or what was defined as a sufficient supply of sewerage). To read a sanitary map was to measure the distance between the mapped space and the ideal, and as sanitary maps were drafted with attention to remediation of urban problems, it was also to envision a method and a narrative of progress: so many months of resewering, so many slums cleared, so many streets drained.

MAPS AS INFORMATION

All maps are rhetorical. That is, all maps organize information according to systems of priority and thus, in effect, operate as arguments, presenting only partial views, which construct rather than simply describe an object of knowledge. Most maps flatten the terrain, offering a view of space as homogenous and equivalent. Maps rarely account for many aspects of time, differences between day and night or the seasons. Human activity, in all its many forms, organizes the terrain in other ways often difficult to represent with conventional cartographic symbols (although in the twentieth century great strides have been made). In any case, these constraints don't make for bad maps, only, inevitably, ones limited by the purposes for which they are intended and the uses to which they are put. Thematic maps, as a subset of maps generally and especially as statistical arguments, are inevitably persuasive in intent.

However, maps, much like anatomy, have generally been accorded a disproportionate truth value by their readers, and often even by their makers, who should know better. Like the body, the earth seems the very stuff of materiality, the privileged referent of truth and experience. Maps, of all documents, are often read uncritically as representations of an external reality, not subject to a platonic distrust of language. As Edney observes,

> The scientific gaze claims to be a naturalistic gaze which . . . creates "topographical drawings." The ability to make [these] . . . , to portray physical fea-

tures in a precise and correct manner . . . was an ability expected of any well-educated individual of the upper classes [in the mid-nineteenth century]. . . . The first superintendent of the British Royal Military College (founded in 1799) held that "everything which is put down in writing of necessity takes on some colour from the opinion of the writer. *A sketch map allows of no opinion.*" (55, original emphasis)

The faith of the average man in maps was sufficiently widespread for Dickens to lampoon it; as we saw in the preface, young Martin Chuzzlewit is so impressed by a plan of the North American city of Eden that, despite the fact that he knows it is not all built, he believes it to be "really a most important place!" (355).

Social problems, including epidemic disease, crime, and prostitution, were seen as especially attendant on urbanization. London and Paris drew particular attention from cartographers and those interested in social work who set about to determine the spatial relations of such problems. Maps of "moral statistics," which began to be popular in France beginning with the first choropleth map in 1826, were well known in England and began to be produced there by the 1830s (Robinson, *Early Thematic Mapping*). Social maps of crime and moral turpitude of various sorts were quite popular, and poverty maps led to the well-known verbal and cartographic mappings of London by Mayhew (maps published in 1862) and Booth (1889). Sanitary reports, of course, included many detailed maps to show the location of nuisances; most of these were pragmatic (at such and such a place, a drain is wanted), but many were intended to be persuasive. Some were used for persuasive purposes in publications addressed to a larger audience, such as Chadwick's report maps of 1842, drawn by Baker. The availability of general-purpose maps made thematic and medical mapping much easier for the medic or sanitarian without expertise in cartography. In the 1890s the Booth maps, for example, were created by researchers in the field who added seven colors showing degrees of poverty to existing Ordinance Survey maps. They then sent them to the publisher, Stanford, who overprinted the colors on his six-inch map of London, "Stanford's library map of London and its suburbs" (J. Elliot 78).

Jarcho argues that early disease maps (before 1840) developed mapping techniques as follows: identification of places, then places with dates and lines of spread, then affected regions in solid colors ("Yellow Fever" 137)—he forgets spot maps in this summary—which he argues shows a "trend toward complexity" (137). This is a questionable conclusion. The definition of complexity is unclear. What is clear from looking at all the maps that Jarcho, E. W. Gilbert, and Stevenson examine, plus some that none discuss in detail (such as the world cholera maps), is that the trajectory of mapping in medical writing, at least as regards cholera, generally moved away from models which showed lines of spread to models that highlighted locality, especially, in medical analyses, spot maps, and from larger views (India, Asia, the world) to smaller views (Oxford, London, Broad St., and Golden Square). However, even this is not a direct line of development, since very localized spot maps were used (for example, Seaman's in 1796—see Stevenson) in the United States for yellow fever, and world and continental maps continued to show up in the 1860s and 1870s. Although historians of cartography, especially in the 1960s and 1970s, repeatedly attempt to show a teleology from simple to complex, the facts rarely bear this out. In fact, all the significant techniques of thematic mapping used well into the twentieth century evolved very rapidly, and were in use by the early to mid-nineteenth century—and with sufficient publicity to ensure that they were widely known.

So we must look elsewhere to explain the choices made by medical mappers. Stevenson is the only historian I have found who sustains a reading of medical maps as arguments. In his study of early yellow fever spot maps, he finds that they tended to be used to make anticontagionist arguments. The history of contagionism and anticontagionism is complex as each of these positions actually embraced many medical theories. However, in broad terms, we can define these here as the positions supporting direct human spread of the cholera versus those who believed epidemics spread by some other means, perhaps climatic. Sanitarians, as believing that disease was caused by filth rather than contact with the sick, fell largely, if problematically, into the anticontagionist camp. Anticontagionism, a stance that, not incidentally, supported commercial interests that would have been damaged by quarantines, was arguably the dominant medical paradigm in the 1830s. Yet, it required constant defense against a popular common sense that "the Fever" (a large category of disease under which cholera was often subsumed by medics and laypeople alike) was contagious.[15] Stevenson discusses several spot maps, which often map incidences of fever against nuisances, which show anticontagionist arguments (for example, the 1920 map by Middleton that shows cases of illness ashore in the harbor, but doesn't include cases on shipboard because of their foreign origin! [244]). Stevenson argued that the spot map was best used for statistical arguments of extreme localism, most often by anticontagionists "of strong sanitarian proclivities" (248), though later contagionists also took them up, perhaps in part because their earlier use in texts that the contagionists wished to refute set the terms of the genre.

Of course the most famous medical map of the period, Snow's Broad Street map, is precisely both antisanitarian and a spot map. (It argued for human spread of cholera, not through direct contact, but through the fecal oral route via contaminated water.) Still, contagionist uses, according to Stevenson, are rare. Stevenson also notes, as few other historians of medical maps do, that these maps were ancillary materials used to prove a thesis, not research tools in themselves. (Stevenson also remarks that medical maps were not used by those interested in atmospheric abnormalities because they "had no way to use it." Although true of local maps, this is in no way self-evident in the case of large-scale maps, such as the world maps showing lines of spread. In fact, as we shall see, Robert Lawson used a world map for a similar purpose. Such maps were much more useful in contagionist arguments.) A great deal of attention was paid to atmospheric and meteorological conditions, and we are now finding that the Victorian interest in such things may not have been so daft. Recent work shows that temperature changes in the sea may have a great impact on cholera epidemics and that the human gut is not the only reservoir of cholera vibrios, as previously believed, but that the vibrios may remain in an inactive state in water for some time before being activated by environmental conditions.

In short, we cannot simply look to a natural progression of increasingly complex means of representation becoming available, and therefore, being used. Medical mappers chose their techniques based on a wide variety of reasons, ranging from a self-conscious decision to choose the mode which favored their argument to simple imitation of existing maps to which they were responsive. As this would suggest, mapmakers did not design these maps in a vacuum, but often related to existing maps and narratives intertextually. Whether they were simply responding to the requirements of a governing body demanding certain kinds of information and protocols for representing them, or responding to the assertions of a rival theorist, mapmakers' choices were more influenced by policy and argumentative aims than technical innovations. But as we shall see, maps did change over time, not to reflect more sophisticated techniques in mapmaking, but to intertextually acknowledge an existing map literature and to reflect political and historical trends which were not, in themselves, cartographic. Increasing reliance on an existing series of mapping documents did enable an increasingly complex and layered historical account of space—for example, showing the changing patterns of disease distribution over time—which encouraged the incorporation of geographic change into narratives of progress.

Biostatistics, putatively objective numbers about corporeal bodies, and maps, objective representations of terra firma, were a perfect match—scientific, based in mathematics and material reality, unanswerable. As Mary Poovey points out, "[N]umbers have come to epitomize the modern fact, because they have come to seem preinterpretive or even somehow noninterpretive even as they have become the bedrock of modern systematic knowledge" *(History of the Modern Fact,* xii), a definition of the notion of the fact which she demonstrates was largely in place by the early nineteenth century, though certainly still not uncontested.[16] Cartography also seemed to inhabit this realm of the absolute and atheoretical. Nor has this trusting attitude significantly altered. As late as

1989, J. B. Harley famously called for an interpretive study of cartography rooted in social theory: against cartographers' claims that maps are mirrors of nature, Harley argued that cartographic vocabulary "embodies a systematic social inequality. The distinctions of class and power are engineered, reified and legitimated in the map by means of cartographic signs" (7) and naturalized by a discursive mindset in which "science itself becomes the metaphor . . . for a utilitarian philosophy and its will to power" (10). Writing specifically of medical maps in 1980, distinguished expert in medical geography G. M. Howe warns:

> [S]ince maps may be read, used, and acted upon by other professions [than cartography], it is of the utmost importance that their limitations and total dependence on the quality of the data be realized. Otherwise an impression of totally spurious reliability may be conveyed. . . . [T]here is no single epidemiological index which completely characterizes the impact of a disease in a community. . . . Maps or cartograms explain nothing but they all pose the question "Why?" This inevitably leads to a search for explanations of the spatial patterns revealed [which must take into account many complex factors]. (284–85)

Howe, whose work is largely of the type medical geographers today would call "positivist," still emphasizes the contingent and partial nature of the knowledge produced by medical mapping, as well as underscoring most readers' naïveté regarding the status of this knowledge.

But many other late-twentieth-century medical cartographers and historians are less cautious. For example, in a passage which has been widely and uncritically reproduced, Thrower enthuses that Snow's 1855 maps "illustrate the highest use of cartography: to find out by mapping that which cannot be discovered by other means" (*Maps and Civilization* 152)—despite the fact that Snow created the Broad Street map after he had already reached his conclusions, in order to illustrate them persuasively. (The maps were not even published until the second edition of his paper on the Golden Square outbreak.) As we will see, there is nothing natural about the way Snow chose to construct his maps, not to test a hypothesis, but to argue a thesis. Additionally, modern cartography is historically complicit with and driven by imperialist and capitalist expansion. Between some sense of map as ideal and territory as real, which many critics of maps assume, there is Geoff King's articulation of the Marxist position that materiality and ideal are not separable. Mapping creates a territory, and certainly participates in the creation of place, in the sense that mapping often determines or alters the human practices within the territory it defines: "Capitalism can be seen as an amalgam of map and territory, a complex and multifaceted series of mutually reinforcing structures that maintain its now almost global hegemony" (King 168).

This is especially obvious in the case of plans, which map future environments and partially create their conditions of possibility. Yet it is true of existing maps as well, which act to limit future interactions with an existing environment, as well as fixing it politically and legally, for example, through zoning laws, constituency definitions, and so forth. Although some historical maps have begun to receive this kind of scrutiny (most notably Renaissance maps of the New World), nineteenth-century sanitary and medical maps have been accorded no such attention. Yet these maps played a significant part in establishing the spatial discourse of the social body and in shaping the Victorian sense of how cities work, a set of beliefs which still resonate in urbanism today.

In human geography, which focuses on human practices of space and of which medical geography is a part, there have been, over recent years, increasingly insistent calls for attention to place over space. If space is the Euclidean description of a site's physical properties and relation to other sites, place takes into account the ways in which human beings use space to construct meaningful referents and sites for human activity—again, what Lefebvre and other theorists have called "social space." Place includes the practical, emotional, and economic qualities of human interactions with space, among other aspects. Humanist, feminist, and postmodern geographers have been loudest in their calls for mapping place, which includes chronological elements of human interaction as well, and pays attention to identity, including gender, class, and race/ethnicity, as well as agency as issues in the practice of space. The WHO's challenging definition of health as "a state of complete physical, mental, and social well-being and not merely the absence of disease" (1) has pushed medical geographers to move to more holistic, complex measures of health than earlier foci simply on disease incidence or mortality.

However, even as recently as 1994, Robin Kearns's call for an integration of social and medical geography was met with incomprehension from environmental determinists Mayer and Meade. It is not surprising, then, that when medical geography was in its Enlightenment era infancy, it should have concerned itself with what we might consider a positivist approach. Although historians of medical geography trace its lineage back to Hippocrates' *De Aere, Aquis et Locis,* as Howe has noted, until germ theory, emphasis was on the internal balance of the body rather than external causes (282). However, epidemic disease in the age of world transportation was able to draw attention to environmental factors even in the early nineteenth century, long before germ theory gained currency. Although some very early maps of plague and the like sporadically appeared very early, serious attention to medical topography with cartography seems to have begun around 1810 (E. W. Gilbert). By 1840, the number of cholera maps extant has been described as "intractably large" to address in any one study (Jarcho, "Yellow Fever" 131).

Medical topography became an important part of place definition, with policy and economic ramifications. E. W. Gilbert notes that when, "in his book on climate, Dr. Clark praised the then unknown Ventnor in the Isle of Wight as a health-giving winter resort; his commendations sent up the price of building land [. . .] from £100 per acre to £800 or £1000 in a very few years" (173). Mapping also became an important part of professionalism. In the United States, maps were considered so important that the first law for copyright protection was created in 1790, "for the Encouragement of Learning, by securing the Copies of Maps, Charts and Books to the Authors and Proprietors" (qtd. in Stevenson 237). (Plagiarism was still sufficiently lucrative worldwide for Berghaus to complain about it in the preface to his Atlas in the late 1840s.)

Robinson demonstrates that maps were in widespread use among the educated classes by midcentury; to ignore the mapping trend was to be out of step with the times. Joseph Fletcher, a moral statistician, published his 1847 paper on educational and moral statistics with "one simple reference map," observing that the tables were as expressive as "an expensive series of shaded maps" (qtd. in Robinson, *Early Thematic Mapping* 162). Robinson observes, however, "His anticartographic attitude soon did an about-face. Only two years later, in 1849, he published another study . . . accompanied by twelve relatively elaborate maps." He explained, "A set of shaded maps accompanies these tables . . . I have endeavored to supply the deficiency which H.R.H. Prince Albert was pleased to point out, of the want of more illustrations of this kind" (qtd. in Robinson, *Early Thematic Mapping* 162). As Robinson mentions, it is significant that when Petermann (later "Physical Geographer and Engraver on Stone to the Queen," E. W. Gilbert 178) first sought to establish himself in England, he began with medical maps, specifically of cholera in the British Isles. This shows the importance such maps had in the period (Robinson, *Early Thematic Mapping* 177).

It would be overstating the case to assert that medical maps were the primary thematic concern of cartographers in this period. But they were a type of map most interesting to those in the medical profession, who not only constructed but also perused them, to sanitarians, to local boards, and to some extent to the general public, at least during and immediately after an epidemic. Medical maps, then, created an interest and a public disproportionate to their merits as aesthetic or technical artifacts. In recalling attention to these maps and attempting to read them, not simply as positivist representations of the land which are more or less flawed by the scientific resources which mapmakers had, but as cultural documents in dialogue with other narratives, beliefs, and ideological investments, I am gesturing toward the social space—perceived and conceived—that these maps both encode and attempt to change.

Restoration of a sense of lived space to these maps is extremely difficult. However, it is possible to view these maps critically, examining what they chose to do and not to do and what investments they may have represented. It is also possible to reconstruct some circumstances of their reception, as we shall see in chapter 4. Although this is only a first step toward understanding the role these maps might have played in constructing perceptions of space, it is a necessary one—and long overdue. After a flurry of attention in the 1960s and 1970s, which consisted mostly of simply noting the existence of such maps and forming a chronology of their production, little has been done with these representations. Outside of Lloyd Stevenson's 1965 article on early yellow fever spot maps, there has been no sustained attention to the rhetorical nature and context of their production. Additionally, map historians tend to be most fascinated with maps which display technical innovation, whereas our purpose here is better met by examining maps which chart the thematic interests of the medical profession and were fairly widely disseminated.

In light of these facts, I shall discuss here a number of maps that have not been examined before, as well as some that have. These maps, of course, were not published or consumed in a vacuum; they were accompanied by textual reports. I shall read them in that context, sampling also other narratives of perceived space that affected both their construction and reception. In chapter 5, we will examine an exemplary novel, Dickens's *Bleak House*, which both responds to these maps and attempts the same act of representation: that is, to show a difference between perceived and conceived space and relate the bridging of that difference to narratives of liberal development. But whereas the texts have received considerable attention from political, literary, and medical historians over the years, the maps, which were a significant part of the production of both knowledge and visual culture in this period, have not, and it is to that end that I emphasize them proportionately here. The principal contribution of this volume is intended to be not a comprehensive reading of these documents, which would be beyond the scope of any one study, but to gesture toward how important such documents were in producing some of the spatialized discourse of the social body in the period and to contextualize and interpret documents which have too long been either ignored or, worse, left unchallenged as transparent records of "fact"—and because "factual," ahistorical.

PART II

Mapping Disease
in the Metropole

2

Visible at a Glance

English Sanitary and Medical Maps

When the 211 deaths are mapped upon a houseplan of the City (as may conveniently be done by stamping a black ink mark at each place where one of these has occurred) the broad features of the epidemic will be visible at a glance. . . . [T]heir distribution may be noticed especially in two directions: many, dotted about in confined and crowded courts, where domestic cleanliness is rare, and atmospheric purity impossible; many, on the southern slope of the City, where it is a habitual complaint that stenches arise from the sewers.

> —John Simon, *Report on the Cholera Epidemic of 1854 as it Prevailed in the City of London*

Sound national health and sanitation has been said to be that physical condition of a nation which enables the individuals composing it to discharge rightly their respective functions in the State. . . . Sanitation is the attempt to influence for good by all known methods the factors which bear on the national health; to promote education in its truest sense, physical, intellectual and moral.

> —Henry W. Acland, "The Influence of Social and Sanitary Conditions on Religion"

AS FOUCAULT, DONZELOT, POOVEY and others have suggested, the nineteenth century was obsessed with visibility. The city, in particular, became subject to a

27

scrutiny which was as much devoted to actively establishing transparency as it was to simply recording what was already present. Modes of knowing[1] devoted to understanding the urban social body, especially its poor and sick, which tabulated and described them and their ways of life, were also devoted to managing them. District visitors not only surveyed the poor, gathering information, but intervened in the lives of the visited. The information they and medics gathered was made into charts and graphs, was analyzed statistically—and mapped. "Sweetness and light"—that is, fresh air and sunlight, both indicative of the openness and circulation that was rarely found in the crowded courts and lodging houses of the urban poor, became in the 1860s a metaphor for Arnoldian culture and civilization, but began as a very literal requirement of public health. This openness, of course, also enabled the poor to be seen. The *savoirs* of the social were emphatically visual genres, and if the verbal descriptions of the poor and sick were replete with metaphors of invisibility, foreignness, barbarity, and darkness, as Peter Keating, among others, has suggested, then the emerging social sciences promised confidently to shed light on the urban social body, rendering it visible at a glance, and thus available for intervention and civilization. In the face of a space perceived as opaque and corrupt, social theorists conceived a space which would be transparent, in which individual bodies would be evenly distributed and behave in predictable ways which would continue to enhance their visibility.

Medics and sanitarians—overlapping but not necessarily identical groups—became part of the knowledge system of professional social management.[2] Scientific knowledge increasingly supplemented and sometimes supplanted more traditional modes of authority. Medics, in particular, came into prominence as a profession which, as certain health issues became public issues, for the first time had a significant role to play in social governance. As they prescribed for populations, instead of individuals, spatial knowledge became an increasingly important part of the medic's toolkit. Traditional medical geography, extending back to Hippocrates, combined with the new statistical sciences to give authority to the medic as specifically public figure, and the disease map became an important part of that authority. As early sanitary maps of nuisances gave place to increasingly sophisticated maps which claimed a specifically medical knowledge as a source of authority, these maps increasingly referenced a palimpsestic model of space which used historical changes in the environment in a narrative of progress. As the midcentury arrived, that narrative of sanitary progress was increasingly tied to another narrative which permeated liberal discourse of the time—one of national development out of the mists of barbarism towards the ideal of civilization.

Sanitary and medical maps contributed to a redefinition of community as a spatial entity centered around the body and the built and natural environment. Local reports on sanitary conditions of large towns began to be generated under the Health of Towns Inquiry in the mid-1840s. A substantial minority—perhaps a quarter to a third—of these were accompanied by maps, and often by more than one.[3] Of the local sanitary reports to the General Board of Health published mostly between 1849 and 1854 under the Public Health Act in response to the upcoming cholera epidemic, it must be said that they vary tremendously. (They also often cover much smaller communities than the earlier Health of Towns inquiry.) But they are, only a few years after the earlier reports, now usually accompanied by a map, and sometimes several. The General Board appears to have asked for accounts of sewerage, drainage, supply of water, and general sanitary condition of inhabitants. In response, the text may be quite brief, or prolix; the map may be a simple map of the area, or it may show every nuisance, or housing diagrams, or sewerage, or even plans for sanitary amendments.

All towns seem to have held public meetings on the topic, and the report had to be publicly available in case anyone wanted to send amendments to the general board. Often such reports and amendments have to do with drawing or redrawing the boundaries of a district, which in itself might go far toward reconceiving space, and as this involved the ratepayers in responsibility for any space included, these concepts of community were sometimes hotly contested. This is evident in William Rider's report on the parish of Haworth, to take a random example, wherein ratepayers objected to a plan to annex part of Oxenhope to Haworth for sanitary purposes. The annexation was based on the supposed dependency of the part of Oxenhope on Haworth for drainage and its abutment on Haworth on a main road; in terms of sewerage, the argument ran, they should be—and would be—connected. The objection was based, apparently, both on a financial argument of disproportionate burden by the ratepayers and also on their sense that they really were separate communities with different characteristics and values, despite their proximity.

Here one sees an understanding of community which begins to shift from one based on the self-concept of residents formed around traditional and legal parish boundary definitions and residents' practice of space, to one concerned with the interdependence of geographic features (and their sanitary implications) and the bodies and bodily functions of residents— thus inaugurating a new concept and, potentially, a new practice of space. The redefinition of a community to include a neighboring community based on its sanitation would create new financial obligations, new relationships, (perhaps initially of intolerance and hostility to the newly incorporated, less affluent community) new building opportunities—in short, create a new legal entity which in turn would encourage a renegotiation and transformation of the built environment. Whether a given community was legally redefined or not, the process of arguing out the implications forced at least community leaders to think through other ways of defining the spaces they practiced than those traditionally used.

Sanitary mapping could be done by medics or laymen, since it relied on the common sense perception of unpleasant smells and visible dirt. It is important here to keep in mind the connections Victorians made between disease, morality and the body. As we have seen, for Victorians, epidemic disease was a sign of poor sanitary practices which were tied to poor economic and moral practices; in turn dirt caused immorality, by so violating the boundaries of the body and psyche as to degrade the self's tenuous ability to preserve independence from its surroundings, human and inanimate. Especially under the early sanitary movement of Chadwick, from the late 1840s through the mid-1850s, filth, to be carefully mapped onto the urban terrain preparatory to intervention, was an index of moral corruption on the body social and in the individual bodies that comprised it. This index was clear to any person of ordinary abilities who understood where to look. Excise the filth from the civic body, it was reasoned, and the health of the social body must follow. In this way, the individual humans who lived in slums were, by those who represented the city to the sanitary establishment in maps, drained of agency, massified, and mapped as inert, usually dark areas, whether representing epidemic deaths or simply filthy slums, onto a city whose body would respond to treatment.

As the century wore on and gains were made in the most basic levels of sanitation—the improvement of sewerage and so forth—medical mapping and sanitary mapping, which later devolved back into social mapping, begins to split off, though they still overlap. Medical mapping begins to suggest more sophisticated, hidden relationships between geography, the built environment, and disease that only the doctor and sanitary engineer can interpret. On the other hand, social geographers find that poverty and social ills cannot simply be reduced to a one-to-one relationship with deleterious places; there came to be understood a complex and dynamic relationship between places, what was seen as inadequate social practice, and the organic functions of growth in a great city. Finally, however, social geographers continued to be heavily influenced by medical mapping's increasing tendency to represent urban spaces anatomically, eliding individual bodies in a representation of the large, passive body of the city which required a medicalized intervention. Obviously, there was a good deal of overlap between these concepts and the progression is not an unproblematically linear one. But as a broad outline of urban social geography's development in this period, it is reasonably accurate. To suggest a sense of this progression, the following two chapters will look at, in turn, English social and sanitary mapping, especially that related to the cholera, in the first half of the century, and at John Snow's groundbreaking work on cholera and the immediate responses to it which marked an era of increasing medicalization of the community and the city.

THE SANITARY PROJECT: GAVIN

The comprehensive mapping of health in England was initiated under the
sanitary project of Edwin Chadwick, which mapped both individual epidemics and generally unhealthy places (that is, those with accumulations of
filth). Many of the most widely perused sanitary maps were accompanied by
text and statistics, and circulated in pamphlet form. Hector Gavin's 1848
pamphlet, based on data gathered in the service of Chadwick's sanitary project, was published separately from his findings in the Sanitary Reports. It was
apparently intended for a more general audience of middle-class elites bent on
social improvement and perhaps charity, though it may not have circulated
very widely. Titled *Sanitary Ramblings, being . . . sketches and illustrations of
Bethnal Green, a Type of the Condition of the Metropolis,* it is an excellent example of a convergence of discourses on the city. "Ramblings" places it in a tradition of guidebook literature, pleasant guides to picturesque walks, except, of
course, here the picturesqueness is ironically alluded to. The sketches and
illustrations are both visual and verbal; detailed sanitary narratives tend to go
district by district, beginning with an overview and then proceeding street by
street and court by court, and Gavin follows this model. There are also two
maps, one showing sewers and open sewers and the other showing sewers and
using variable shading to indicate the location of "cholera mist" in Bethnal
Green. The argument is entirely sanitary; that is, it connects mortality and
morbidity to cleanliness. Dirt represents poverty, and comes to stand in for
economic deprivation. Dirt was a solvable problem.

Gavin originally wrote his report for Chadwick's Board Report, which
quotes it extensively but does not include it all; perhaps this also influenced
his decision to bring it out separately. Among other points he makes that do
not appear in the Chadwick report is that the "middle and upper classes" are
the ones that "really cause" the "neglect of cleanliness" which destroy the lives
of the poor (79), a statement which Chadwick may have thought impolitic in
its bluntness. As Christopher Hamlin points out in his excellent study, as the
architect of the New Poor Law, Chadwick was highly motivated to elide "want
of the necessaries of life" as a cause of disease, an elision against which the
medics working under him sometimes rebelled. Although many of the people
working under Chadwick had no medical training, Hector Gavin was in fact
a doctor. However, within the sanitary model, medical training was beside the
point—anyone in the possession of one's senses, Chadwick assumed, could
manage to identify the bad smells and visible filth which caused disease.

Gavin's use of graphics displays the uneasy transition between an earlier
use of illustration as exemplary and the newer, scientific emphasis on mimesis.
In addition to the maps, for example, Gavin uses a woodcut from the pages of
the *Poor Man's Guardian* which shows the overcrowded condition of a lodging

house in cross section. This, he says, will do to show the perniciousness of inns and such—although he admits that Bethnal Green in fact has no lodging houses (68)! Here we see the tension between kinds of representation; the text and map depend on their specificity and eyewitness empiricism (see fig. 2.1). But Gavin's point is precisely that Bethnal Green is a "type" as he says in the title, and thus a fictitious woodcut will do as well as anything drawn from the actual place (as, for example, Mayhew claims to have in his illustrations, although many of the drawings were actually heavily typological). The unique, scientific map and the general impressionistic sketch come together: like the "wavy lines" to represent rivers (see chapter 1, p. 12), irrespective of any actual changes in the watercourse at that level of detail, the sketch represents with broad accuracy the specific details contained in the narrative, which themselves

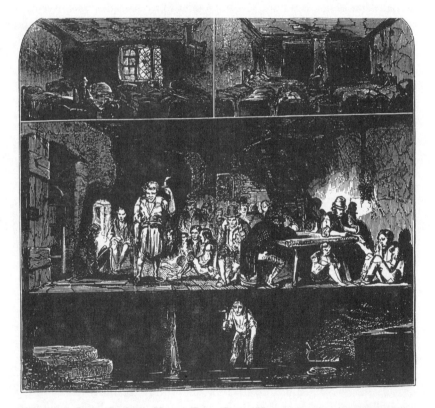

FIGURE 2.1. Gavin: Lodging House. From Gavin, Hector. *Sanitary Ramblings. Being Sketches and Illustrations of Bethnal Green. A Type of the Condition of the Metropolis and other Large Towns.* London: J. Churchill, 1848.

are hardly very specific except as to place name and address (after all, how many hundreds of houses had been described, by this time, as "indescribably filthy ... with family members sleeping together promiscuously"?).

This is precisely the tense contradiction that balances to create realism in fiction: the specific example must be individual, yet represent a type general enough to be recognized within generic conventions and also mobilize a wider appeal. A river that ran straight would look like a "wire," and so must not be represented that way regardless of its true direction. Still, the map legitimates its narrative with the illusion of absolute specificity and transparency. This, too, is the logic of statistical representation. The individual statistic must be an accurate description of a single, supposedly unique instance, yet must have applicability within a standardized framework; it must indicate something more than its own specificity. For these conditions to be attained, there must be a sense of a large category of objects whose specific differences are less significant than their common features. Under liberal economic theory, such a common feature might be the tendency of purchasers to pay the lowest price for goods. The body became that unit of structural equality for social theorists, subject to uniform rules regarding proximity to wastes, to other bodies, and so forth, the violation of which resulted in predictable social ills.

But the maps here are more than a scientific representation of a specific physical phenomenon or even of an abstract theory; they also serve a narratological function. The text is bracketed by two maps: the one at the beginning, which marks out open sewers in strong black lines and the closed ones in double thin lines, and the map at the end, under which the details of the lines representing the terrain are just visible in areas heavily shaded by "cholera mist" (see figs. 2.2 and 2.3). The threatening dark shading of the mist represents a spiritual blight:

> [T]he accompanying lithographic plate of the parish exhibits the Disease Mist . . . ; the Angel of death *[sic]* not only breathes pestilence, and causes an afflicted people to render back dust for dust, but is accompanied with that destroying Angel which breathes a moral pestilence; for where the seeds of physical death are abundantly sown, and yield an abundant harvest, there moral death overshadows the land,—and sweep with the besom of destruction to an eternal gulf! (Gavin 101)

The people are mapped onto the land as soil for a harvest of disease and sin, and then are swept entirely off the map into hell in this dramatic passage. It also visibly represents invisibility—in Milton's phrase, "darkness visible"—both in the cholera mist and in the dramatization of the obscurity under which Bethnal Green labors. If it can be seen and represented, it can be saved. Gavin opens his pamphlet with the following quote from the Health of Towns Reports and then explains his reasons for publishing:

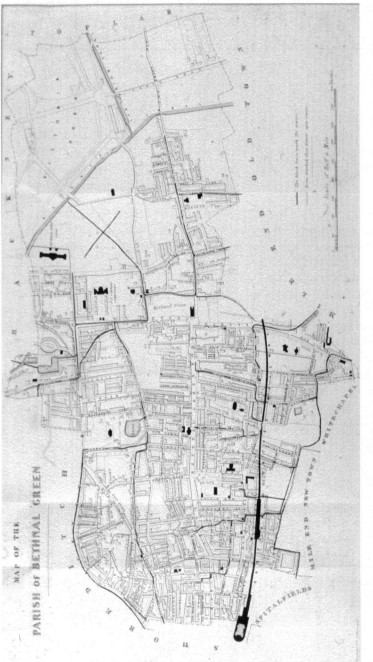

FIGURE 2.2. Gavin: Bethnal Green. From Gavin, Hector. *Sanitary Ramblings. Being Sketches and Illustrations of Bethnal Green. A Type of the Condition of the Metropolis and other Large Towns.* London: J. Churchill, 1848.

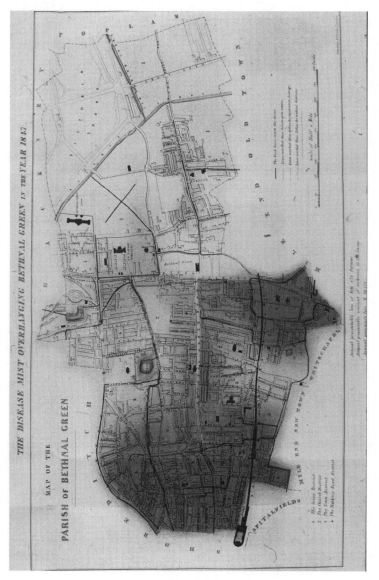

FIGURE 2.3. Gavin: Bethnal Green with Disease Mist. From Gavin, Hector. *Sanitary Ramblings. Being Sketches and Illustrations of Bethnal Green. A Type of the Condition of the Metropolis and other Large Towns.* London: J. Churchill, 1848.

"Owing to the vastness of London," says Mr. Martin [in the Health of Towns Report], "owing to the moral gulf which there separates the various classes of its inhabitants—its several quarters may be designated as assemblages of towns rather than as one city; and so it is in a social sense, and on a smaller scale, in other towns; *the rich know nothing of the poor;* the mass of misery that festers beneath the affluence of London and of the great towns is not known to their wealthy occupants." It is true that some partial attempts have been made to display, both locally and generally, many of the remediable ills . . . of London; but no complete elucidation of the sanitary state of any one district has as yet been prominently brought forward for . . . securing the sympathy of the public. (Gavin 4, emphasis in original)

The language is replete with visual metaphors: Gavin will display and elucidate a parish lost in darkness, exemplary of a larger darkness hovering over London and other large towns. The elucidation, or lighting up of the darkness, that is performed by the text is visibly performed by the two maps that border the text. The first map, facing the title page, shows the open and closed sewers. The text inscribes its story of darkness and dirt, street by street, upon the space described by the map. The final map, folding out to face the last page, shows the same image as the first map obscured by sepia "cholera mist."

Gavin concludes the text by observing that no one has taken an interest in or responsibility for the parish: "[T]he very map of the parish, by which its boundaries are ascertained, is (or was a month ago), so tattered, old, and worn, as to be nearly falling to pieces" (Gavin 114). Now that he has written his report and mapped the sanitary and moral condition of the parish, he has cared for it by representing it on a new map. However, the official survey map *is* the parish; its boundaries—preexisting their representation, apparently—cannot be ascertained if the map is allowed to decay. In a pragmatic way, this exemplifies the lack of care for the poor; were anyone actively taking responsibility for this parish, they would be likely to maintain an interest in the boundaries of their burden. But it also indicates an almost metaphysical significance given to the map. The map "ascertains," but it also maintains a community as a parish, with leaders and responsibilities. The neglected map is the neglected community: ragged and ill defined. In fact, Gavin implies, it scarcely is a community anymore at all; as he asks, how can people living in such circumstances believe in brotherly love? It is simply a collection of human and other refuse.

Should the map cease to exist, in some sense, the parish would be finally lost as a community, and as a geographic object of discourse and intervention. As the map turns to waste paper, the people are in danger of being swept away, by that "besom of destruction," unregarded. This also implies that the map is out of date, that places (houses, people) are, quite literally, "off the map," which again implies a lack of community care and an obligation to go, map in hand, and look at the terrain represented, remapping and reinscribing it. In Chadwick's sanitary model, anyone with common sense, a good nose, and ordinary vision could see and map the degenerate social and urban body.

The first map attempts a certain transparency; it invites readers to go, look for themselves, and see exactly what the map shows. The mist which obscures the terrain delineated below it dramatizes the obscurity of the unmapped parish in its moral benightedness. At the same time, as Gavin repeatedly has cause to mention, the map freezes a moment in time, whereas sanitary conditions are constantly changing. He observes that due to an earlier lecture that he gave, some conditions have been remedied, but others have sprung up. If the first map defines at least a situation of some duration—current locations of sewers are unapt to change overnight—the second map defines a moment in time, as "mist" is nothing if not mobile with the winds and wholly evaporates in a short period, although this mist is defined as lasting and persistently clinging to the low-lying areas near the open drains. In that sense, the second map is not transparent, since it is impossible to go and see "the disease mist," but points to a temporary situation which will recur without radical emendations to the first map.

The parish should know its condition, and the medium through which that knowledge is produced is the map; the map makes visible the illness of the city. Abstract representation is the mode by which the city can be produced as object of knowledge and, in turn, managed so as to perpetuate itself along the lines prescribed for it—to become more like the ideal mapping, fitting itself into a grid of manageability. Like a surgical diagram, the map shows illness as a dark sepia obscurity on the otherwise healthy body of the city, preparatory to a surgical excision. If Gavin's mapping invokes the coherent fate of an inadequately socialized social body, it also dramatizes the need to continually remap its terrain in order to arrest decadence and record or invoke progress. Sanitary writers urge a continual vigilance—to look, and document, and look, and look again, as to lose sight of, or fail to oversee, a problematic district is precisely to lose control of it, to allow it to disintegrate or degenerate into that sea of wastes which forever besets the integrity of the social body.

General sanitary mapping peaks in the midcentury, especially from 1849 to the mid-1860s. Most of these maps were created simply by ordinary gentlemen with minimal training, some by surveyors and engineers, and some (like Gavin's) by medical practitioners. Sanitary maps provided both background information and often the impetus for the cholera maps, which were far more frequently created by medics than by any other category of mapmaker. Indeed, medics stood on their special knowledge as a source of legitimation when creating these maps, even if that special knowledge was merely that of the experience of having treated cholera in a particular community, and the argument of the map was simply a sanitary one. Some of the most fascinating and ultimately useful of these were constructed with an eye to historiography. Thomas Shapter's intriguing history of the 1832 epidemic in Exeter, published on the eve of the second epidemic, has a sanitary argument to support but is primarily intended to be of historical interest, and consequently is full of useful details. In addition to having been an eyewitness of the first epidemic, Shapter goes over historical documents and interviews other eyewitnesses; the result is quite a full and engaging account.

Shapter is anticontagionist and sanitarian, though he gives a good deal of attention to good nutrition as well. He also spends a good deal of space supporting an argument for more financial resources to be allocated to the Board of Health. The map reflects this concern with resources, showing, by the use of numbers, the location of druggists, soup kitchens, and cholera burial grounds, as well as where soiled clothing was burned. Unfortunately, there is no obvious geographic relationship between those resources and mortality, nor does Shapter use the map to try to make such an argument. The map is carefully drawn in black and white, and deaths are marked in red, by the use of one-to-one symbols, which distinguish deaths in 1832, 1833, and 1834 (see fig. 2.4). Shapter observes that the map "has been constructed with great care and attention to particulars, and at the expense of much labour; for I have not only consulted the official returns, the registers of deaths and the registers of burials, but personally and diligently sought information from those engaged in the burials themselves: it thus yields an authentic and curious record of the then state of Exeter" (ix). Curiously, though, he never comments on its significance elsewhere in the text. He is plainly disinterested in using it to advance any particular theory, or as a research tool.

Nonetheless, examination of the map clarifies that it does have a narrative purpose. The map shows the Guildhall, wherein much official business was done, including meetings of the Board of Health; it is also where the members of the medical profession traditionally met and would meet at the end of the narrative to discuss disposal of the gift awarded to them by the grateful authorities, as well as the base of operations for the on-call medics. The Guildhall is one of only three public buildings or landmarks shown on the map that also receive a number, marking it as significant to the narrative. Shapter thus positions both himself and the medical community as professional, and the profession as key to the governmental functions of public health with which the text concerns itself. As to the epidemic, it is enough for his purposes as a historian simply to show the number and location of deaths.

The purpose of this work is not primarily medical, although Shapter uses his status as a doctor to legitimate his authority and, probably, to sell the book. (Thus, in the midst of the historical narrative, there is an oddly anomalous section clinically summarizing the symptoms of cholera and current beliefs about its etiology.) But Shapter's own role as a medical professional is

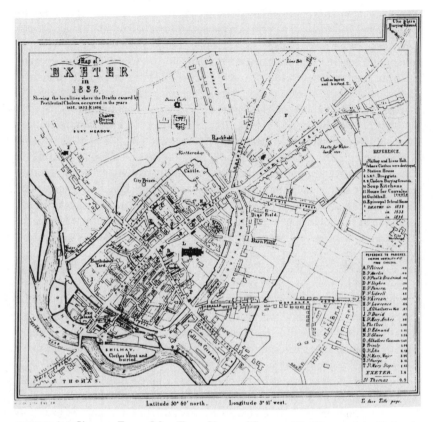

FIGURE 2.4. Shapter: Exeter Map. From Shapter, Thomas. *The History of the Cholera in Exeter in 1832*. London, Churchill, 1849.

key to the narrative, and the narrative itself legitmates medicine as both a profession and a necessary part of government. Shapter's role as a sanitarian, in contrast to many doctors and scientists such as Snow, and as a leading citizen and aficionado of Exeter, complements his Tory identity, and the book is written to consolidate and celebrate his role in the government of the city, in addition to other purposes. In fact, Shapter came to Exeter as a young physician at the age of twenty-four during the cholera outbreak, and was a member of the Chamber, the governing body of Exeter, by 1835 (Newton vi). (Interestingly, again showing his commitment to a simple sanitary rather than medical model, the conservative Shapter, whose connections were with wealthy clergy and professionals, argued in 1870 against improvements under the Health Act of 1858 which were being undertaken to prepare for another cholera epidemic [Newton vi]). Certainly, the cholera epidemic provided an opportunity for medical professionals—already powerful in Exeter (there were seven other physicians in the Chamber in 1835 [Newton vi])—to consolidate their gains, and for Shapter to be quickly noticed as a public citizen. In short, Shapter's book is most interesting as a history of social response to the epidemic and as an example of professional public self-positioning; his map offers little medical information except a sense of how important maps were to that professional self-definition and to readers' constructions of narratives relating to the epidemic.

Shapter's map is representative of a group of specifically historical medical maps and texts produced around this time. There is a clear sense that the 1832 epidemic was an historical event and that there should be historical as well as technical descriptions of it. There is also an emerging professional sense of the importance of case and other medical histories for later research. And finally there is that sense of nostalgia that grips the Victorian writing world for what is perceived as an era that ended with Reform, which we see so clearly in George Eliot's novels. Shapter avows his intention to show what Exeter was like two decades earlier, although now so changed. To that end, not only does the map document topography of a city gone by, but his text is liberally illustrated with woodcuts of the water carriers (an occupation which had disappeared by the time the history was written), old buildings now gone, people disposed in picturesque attitudes and period dress around the main conduit, and so forth (see for example, fig. 2.5, "The Dipping Steps").[4]

Combinations of medical and social history, these texts claim part of their authority as histories on the basis of the clinical eye's observant properties. Woodcuts of slums jockey for space with facsimiles of mortality returns and texts quoted from official correspondence. The map, in its framing position as frontispiece, both contextualizes and provides a spatial field to be inscribed by all that follows. The spatial representation of Exeter, marked with locations of individual deaths, provides the setting upon which we as readers are to inscribe our reading of the narrative that follows. Even the cholera burying ground, set off from the body of both map and referent by an extension of the upper left frame, prepares us for the narrative of its rejection and exclusion by the inhabitants. The map manages to imply that it really isn't part of Exeter (as a square field of space) at all, while simultaneously calling attention to it as a key feature—despite the fact that there is printing room to extend the border of the map across the page, and that placing the border where he does requires that some deaths (on Longbrook Street) must be placed in the border of the map!

The sense of emplotment that placing a disease map in an historical narrative presupposes depends, in these texts, on a mixture of an indulgent sense of nostalgia—in this case for the bygone simplicity and picturesqueness of the

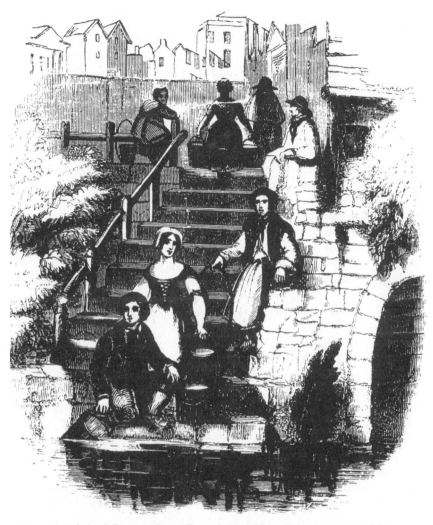

FIGURE 2.5. Acland: Dipping Steps. From Acland, Henry Wentworth. "An Address to the Inhabitants of St. James's, Westminster on certain local circumstances affecting the health of rich and poor." London: James Ridgway, 1847.

working classes of yore and the villagelike qualities of what has since become a substantial urban community. This wistfulness, however, is balanced against the far more common narrative of progress, plotted as a movement away from disorder and superstition and towards lightness, transparency, cleanliness, and science. The index and goal of such progress is health, both moral and physical, which can be read in the cleanliness of the streets and the availability of fresh water. To some extents, these plots balance each other—the loss of the village both necessitates sanitary progress, because of the evils of urbanization, and suggests the modern and therefore desirable possibilities of such development. The fact that what was lovable and aesthetically pleasing about old Exeter is represented as centering around the wells and water conduits drives home the sanitary message and suggests that the aesthetic qualities do not necessarily inhere in village life, but in the cleanliness which will once again be possible with sanitary reform. The historical narrative also emphasizes that change is not only possible but inevitable: conditions are not static, and therefore disease which depends on those conditions is not fated. Shapter involves the geography of the town in a narrative of change and progress—the land is there precisely to be changed in the interest of progress. The vision which looks forward also involves a past, a sense of a community narrative, a mission, and a destiny; the community is the protagonist of this narrative, and Exeter its crucial but malleable setting—and the driving force for change is the medical profession.

ACLAND: PROFESSIONALISM AND THE SOCIAL

Maps beget maps. Once an area had been written about and mapped in connection with cholera, subsequent writers on cholera tended to continue the mapping tradition. It is also the case that those with geographic interests were drawn to literature containing maps and tended then to focus on those areas. It is hardly surprising that Oxford would be one of the places most richly supplied with cartographically minded scholars, and of these, W. P. Ormerod and Henry Wentworth Acland are the most important. Ormerod's 1848 work, coming out contemporaneously with Chadwick's sanitary mappers, is itself a typical sanitary mapping, if unusually detailed, and his dot and shade map distinguished between fever and cholera, but included no dates of onset or directions of spread. His forty-eight-page pamphlet contains an extended mapping narrative from pages 16 to 36, describing dirt, and then analyzing fever mortality; from page 27 until the end, it does the same for cholera without any explicit reference to the map. The map itself is a large foldout, with dots for locations hit by cholera and crosses for places which have suffered fever, but there is no indication of numbers of mortality: that is, a single dot stands for a location in which one or many more may have died. Larger areas (neighborhoods), defined as "the parts chiefly visited by disease generally" are "slightly shaded" (legend). Although he picks out water courses in blue, this appears to be largely an aesthetic move. He does not indicate locations of filth, with which his paper is largely concerned, nor does he comment on the clear trend exposed by the map for disease, in most though not all cases, to follow the water-course, which his blue coloring rather calls attention to.

The map is hand drawn by the author and is quite impressionistic—not to scale, many streets merely suggested, and charming details like trees drawn in to indicate park areas. In short, his detailed charts of deaths by street and date are more useful than the map, and the map itself was apparently more eti-ologically suggestive for his readers than for him. But Acland's excellent 1856 work takes full advantage of the data that Ormerod encodes on his map and then disregards. Of many medics who created maps, many did not know quite what to do with them once they had them, often printing them without com-mentary. However, out of this literature and responding to it arose a new breed of medics who did find uses for such information, who created their own maps and perpetuated a more informed and somewhat more critical tradition, and Acland is one of the finest examples of these. Part of the advantage of this more sophisticated map use is its ability to endow the mapmaker with an authority to speak in the name of the public weal which depends on access to specialized knowledge, one of the hallmarks of professionalism, and Acland makes full use of this authority as well.

Acland's *Memoir* is a beautifully and expensively produced volume, part medical treatise, part history and part social commentary. The ornament of the volume is a large and detailed foldout map at the beginning.[5] He also includes extensive tables of cholera by street of residence and by occupation, in order of date. These are followed by plate 2, a sketch map of Oxford with spots showing places of the first thirty deaths and numbers showing order (see fig. 2.6). Unlike most medics who include sanitary maps without much discussion, Acland repeatedly uses his maps, not merely as illustration, but to prove points. He is a sophisticated map user, as one might expect of a Fellow of the Royal Geo-graphical Society. He urges the reader immediately to compare "Plate 2, or the Sketch Map of Oxford" with his other tables and maps, rather than simply pos-ing it as an illustration sufficient unto itself. He narrates the order and group-ings of deaths and concludes, "[W]e are irresistibly led towards the supposition that Cholera may arise without communication with infected districts on the part of those attacked, but also that it does spread under some circumstances and in some localities from person to person" (21), thus using the map to arrive at, or at least argue for, a conclusion about the cholera's spread, whereas Ormerod's sanitarian paper takes the mode of spread for granted. However, he continues, one needs also to "take a general survey of the [sanitary] condition of the whole Town. For this purpose the Map which is placed at the beginning of the Memoir must be consulted" (21). The map itself has a detailed legend:

Map of Oxford to illustrate Dr. Acland's Memoir on Cholera in Oxford in 1854. Showing the localities in which cholera and choleraic diarrhoea

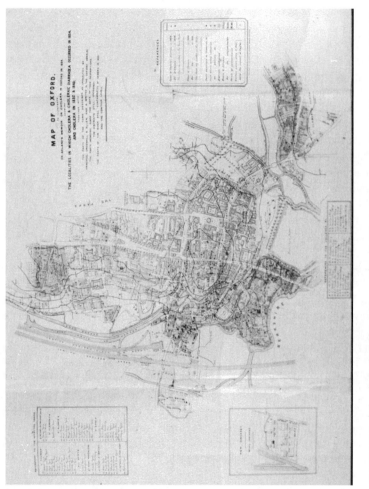

FIGURE 2.6. Acland: Oxford Map. From Acland, Henry Wentworth. "An Address to the Inhabitants of St. James's, Westminster on certain local circumstances affecting the health of rich and poor." London: James Ridgway, 1847.

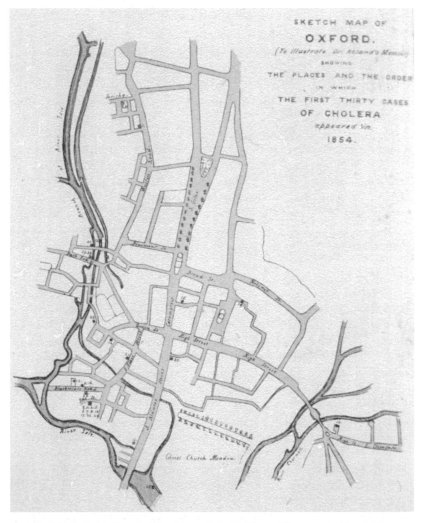

FIGURE 2.7. Acland: Sketch Map. From Acland, Henry Wentworth. "An Address to the Inhabitants of St. James's, Westminster on certain local circumstances affecting the health of rich and poor." London: James Ridgway, 1847.

occurred in 1854, and cholera in 1832 and 1849; together with the parts of the town described as unhealthy, by Ormerod, Greenhill and Allen, and a writer in the Oxford Herald; the parts remedied since the date of their descriptions; the districts still undrained; the parts of the rivers still contaminated by sewers in 1855; and the contour levels. (see fig. 2.7)

Acland refers to Ormerod's map (45),[6] but Acland's map is far more detailed, correctly scaled, and inclusive, incorporating the colleges and St. Thomas parish. He incorporates spot representation of earlier cases on a one-to-one basis, thus giving a sense of relative magnitude of mortality in different areas, and shows an important neighboring parish in a separate box in the margin. The following pages discuss the physical topography of the city and lead the reader through this important and colorful map, which includes contour lines per five feet of elevation and numbers indicating precise elevation. References to the map abound throughout, as he has continual recourse to his investigations on altitude, choosing to study that because the registrar general's report (largely written by William Farr) singled it out as significant. Acland manages a very complex argument in a visually comprehensible and compelling way, in a far more detailed and comprehensive map than Ormerod's, which incorporates the most useful elements of both Ormerod's map and narrative. For example, the map marks by differently shaped "dots" (small rectangles, round dots, and squares) and colors (blue and black) cholera and choleric diarrhoea in 1832, 1849, and 1854, using Ormerod's mapped information about location, but also his narrative information about number of deaths, so as to provide a one-to-one correspondence in a true spot map.[7]

The typical epidemic spot map, as a historical representation, depicts not only space but time.[8] It depicts a span of time—the span of the entire epidemic—as being virtually simultaneous, and has a tendency to concretize, to indicate to the less informed observer that deadly environments are an immutable feature of the terrain depicted. Acland's map, however, attempts to show not only the difference between two different epidemic periods, but between the conditions of nuisances in those two periods. (Still, what remains striking is the depiction of the town near the rivers as enduringly unhealthy.) This is an extremely important development, as it places two epidemics in a continuous narrative over time, the medium of the narrative being spatial; the map becomes a teller of history. Finally, Acland subsequently connects his Oxford to a larger world. Plate 3 shows the area surrounding Oxford and lines of spread from Oxford to surrounding towns. Towns enclosed in an oval had deaths from cholera, towns with double lines extending from Oxford had death(s) "dependent on communication with Oxford" (legend), and those towns whose double line terminates in a star had cholera from Oxford which then spread within the town (see fig. 2.8). It is a sophisticated use of three symbols to signify five variables in a manner visually clear and compelling. It both places Oxford in a regional spatial context and attends to the practice of space by the population—inhabitants of neighboring towns do not remain static in this map; they are engaged in a dynamic of commuting which is represented as an outward movement. Finally, there is another large foldout graphing death rates from cholera.

It is quite clear in looking at the map that deaths in all epidemic periods tend to cluster in roughly the same locations and follow the watercourses, though Acland does not comment on that. It is also clear that the lowest districts near watercourses contaminated with sewage suffer most; the

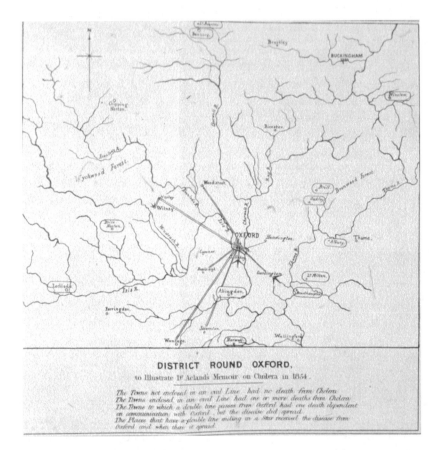

FIGURE 2.8. Acland: District Round Oxford Map. From Acland, Henry Wentworth. "An Address to the Inhabitants of St. James's, Westminster on certain local circumstances affecting the health of rich and poor." London: James Ridgway, 1847.

"undrained" district at the top of the map, which is at a moderate height, suffered somewhat in earlier epidemics, but is untouched in 1854 despite several unremediated nuisances. Certainly this map would support John Snow's theory of a waterborne cholera agent, and Acland was aware of Snow's theory (Acland 77), although he does not find that such contamination can be the sole cause. Acland notes the trend, but attributes it more largely to the *odor* of the contaminated water, though he later remarks

> Mr. Ormerod's Sanitary Map of Oxford points out in an admirable manner the way in which the Epidemic and Contagious Diseases are collected around special centres: and, as may be seen by the Map in this Memoir, these are also about the undrained parts. But I also agree with . . . Mr. Rowell, in the Oxford Journal, Sept. 2, 1854 . . . in districts where the water is impure, the Diseases . . . are the most rife. [W]e cannot reasonably doubt the immediate connection between water and the existence of the disease [in a particular example given]. (51–52)

Acland makes a moderate concession to Snow. It is probably for this reason that he includes the sewage contamination in the map. This is, then, also a good example of a map which by including multiple variables exceeds in usefulness the argument its author intends to portray, and leaves an excess of meaning which is available to interpretation by readers.

To get a sense of the route of spread, we must go to the narrative. Because the "surrounding area" map is a map showing lines of spread, it is much more apparently contagionist than the principal map, which, as a spot map, participates in a sanitarian tradition despite the author's evident sympathy for some kind of contingent or modified contagionist argument. The multipage "Table of Cases of Cholera and Choleraic Diarrhoea in the order of their occurrence" offers a much more powerfully contagionist argument, since addresses are given in the fifth column, and it is clear that they tend to cluster around the same dates in many cases. The sketch map, showing the location and order of the first thirty cases, is the companion piece to this table, and is clearly included to visually render an argument that may be less evident to the reader from the profusion of verbal detail in the table. In the sketch map, nine categories of detail from the chart are eliminated: exact date, sex, age, occupation, result (death or recovery) and date of result (duration), and whether the illness is cholera or choleraic diarrhoea.

Thus, one fails to learn from the map, for example, that the first thirty dead were all laborers, skilled laborers or prisoners, and their wives and daughters (with the exception of a forty-two-year-old architect), or that the mortality was fifty percent, or that the victims ranged in age from five months to seventy-two years, or that only twelve were women, or that only five of those women died, whereas ten of the eighteen men died (despite the fact that in the larger sample of this particular outbreak, more women suffered from cholera and women were also more likely to die). Acland carefully uses both charts and maps to elucidate this kind of data, and mortality by occupation, with breakdown of age, mortality by year and street, meteorology, and so forth, all of which, again, he uses to actually develop the narrative. But in eliminating this data, the spatial relationship of the deaths over the whole epidemic is starkly emphasized on the map in a manner unrepresentable in a chart. Patients, as well, are simplified, homogenized, and abstracted in terms of three significant features of their cases—the fact of their illness, whether the outcome was terminal, and where it took place.

Acland also maps cholera onto the house plans he shows, using numbers to show order and placing the numbers in the space of the room in which the patient dwelt, continuing local mapping at the level of domestic geography. Plate 4 shows plans of tenements and makes a plea for better housing for the poor on the familiar grounds of overcrowding and poisoned air. The plans map cases in order onto the rooms in which they are located (see fig. 2.9). He claims that these tenements are not the worst he could show, nor so badly built, just overcrowded: "This is, in plain words, *life in poisoned air*" (81, emphasis in original). This introduces, in a mapping context, a technique that was to become crucial in later housing literature, of showing the drainage and crowding of houses. Even more importantly, though, it places the cross section of the house in the same context as the mapping of the town: the internal domestic space is a continuation of a larger medical topography and, in turn, affects it.

The carefully maintained division between an Englishman's sovereign domain and the outside world from which it was to be a refuge is eroded, laid bare in a scientific—indeed, anatomical—technique of the cross section which, as D. A. Miller notes of the Victorian novelist, cuts away the walls to allow us to see inside. Yet, unlike the novel, what is revealed is not individuality or subjectivity, but a radical and passive sameness. The tenements are only unique as the site of particular deaths, represented by identical symbols; we see no individualizing detail, and are assured that these are representative homes (just as the body on the postmortem table used to illustrate anatomical texts will later be always assumed to be the representative body). The house plan shows the continuity of the home with the disease, the disease with the town through the home, and by implication, on to the surrounding areas. The individual becomes part of the social body; the home becomes part of the public space of the town, the town of the region, and by extension, the nation, the world.

The idea of space that Acland conveys in the map itself, then, is complex and multilayered—a palimpsest, not only of overlapping time periods, as we see nascent in Shapter, but levels, types, and modes of spatial organization. This palimpsestic mapping indicates connections between the individual and

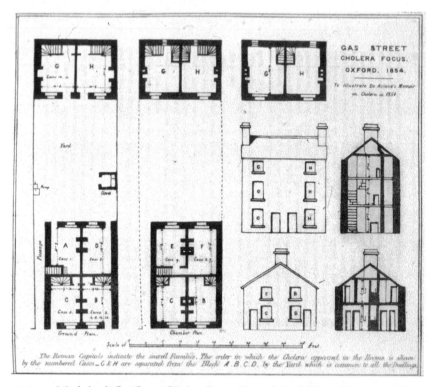

FIGURE 2.9. Acland: Gas Street Cholera Focus. From Acland, Henry Wentworth. "An Address to the Inhabitants of St. James's, Westminster on certain local circumstances affecting the health of rich and poor." London: James Ridgway, 1847.

the larger community, the community and the world, as well as surface and depth, built and natural environments. As space moves to the center of the narrative and becomes more complex, however, the individual is represented increasingly as a passive and interchangeable body afflicted (or not) by geographic circumstance. The narrative in which this space is emplotted is one not only of forward motion through time (and its concommitent inverse allegiances of nostalgia), but of outward motion, from the single to the many, from the individual to the state (and its inverse interpellation of the individual). The emphasis on the circulation of persons between towns emphasizes a responsibility that goes beyond that which is owed to a single parish or community. Thus, the narrative of progress so evident in Acland's text and which underlies most similar publications is imbricated in a complex traversal and retraversal of spaces and levels of spaces, from the birds'-eye view of the area surrounding Oxford to the architectural view of a single home's cross section.

For this view to be depicted—and for it to be meaningful in terms of being implemented—requires a certain standardization of spaces, from a standardized sewerage to a standard organization of houses and their inhabitants (not too many living in a single house, for example). None of this information will have useful predictive value unless people practice the environment appropriately, and that requires a standardization of individual behavior as well.

It is not surprising, given the stakes of this argument, that Acland also claims a social authority within the moral domain. Part 3, "The Lesson of the Epidemic," begins with a rhetoric not dissimilar to that of sermons on the national fast days for the first two cholera epidemics which emphasized the relation between individual responsibility and national sin, though with a sanitary twist:

> Instances of individual self-destruction from avoidable circumstances might be multiplied without end. With these individual cases we have not here to deal. Each man has a free will, and he must make his choice according to the knowledge he possesses. But with communities this is not so: they have law-givers and laws.... [I]t is not to be doubted ... that [civilized] *communities*, as well as *individuals*, may violate the sanitary laws which our Creator has imposed on us; and that the consequence of the violation of these laws is punishment to the *community* for its *common* crime; as it is in the case of the individual for his individual crime.... Life is a holy thing; and if communities throw away the lives of the individuals who compose them, or make these sickly, short and miserable, the community will, in some manner, "pay for it." (105–106, emphasis in original)

There follows a Utilitarian argument about paying rates to support the disabled and orphaned.

Although Acland carefully separates the individual and the community, it seems quite clear from elsewhere in his argument, as he exhorts the sanitary authorities to use their powers to force remediation, that the individual's right to exercise that free will be severely limited when it impacts the larger community. In turn, the community is represented not by a composite of individual wills, but by the more powerful wills of its lawgivers and rulers. Acland's argument evokes the rhetoric of natural laws and general providence, though he stays within the utilitarian rather than the moral rhetoric much of the time. Indeed, it should not be surprising to find language similar to sermons on national sin and disease as punishment, published in response to the first epidemic, here. Medical mapping was often used in the same way that sermons were—to define a community which was inclusive of all classes and which showed the interdependence of the well-to-do reader with the lower classes most likely to suffer from the disease, or be part of the conditions to spread it. In showing the proximity of the streets of high mortality to other areas, medical mapping made a point about community. In identifying communities by district or parish, medical mappers made a point about responsibility.

In his summary of the book's argument, Acland defends the inclusion of the lengthy third section and also its limits in language that evokes England's vision of itself as "civilized" with mild irony:

> It seemed the fitter course . . . to sketch in a broad manner for general consideration certain aspects of Civilized society, as its masses stand in relation to physical and moral causes, in a City which maintains a moderate population. To enumerate the arrangements which a wise Community would adopt beforehand to mitigate the terrible scourge of coming Epidemics, would be to describe the manner in which a civilized and well-regulated people, acquainted with the laws of health and the causes of disease, would strive to live on ordinary occasions: and as this would lead the reader into questions of the most extensive nature—social, so called, political and religious—it cannot be fully discussed in this place. (105)

Acland takes for granted that these questions are social, and that "social" means the relation of the masses to (rather confusingly) "physical and moral causes." England claims to be civilized, but fails to act that way. This argument is formulated, interestingly, in a language of rights, which is, à la T. H. Marshall, connected with childhood: bad water, poor food, inadequate lodgings, bad sanitation, and unventilated schoolrooms make "'the child, the father to the man,' more sickly than he need have been" (Acland 108). That failure to recognize the interconnectedness of the whole community is what is implicitly barbarous:

> The Community may be barbarous or civilized. We have here to do with Civilized Communities only . . . I should be ashamed of dwelling on subjects of this kind, did I not feel that the People of England have yet to awake as from a dream. . . . We must feel the bitterness of the evil which social life entails on the less honourable members of the body politic. The feet must tread the mire, yet they may be clad; and the hands may be washed and warm, though they be thick with toil. It is not simply a wrong to our Fellow Men, if that is withheld which they may justly claim: it is sin and degradation to the Rulers. (105–107)

Having, in fact, adverted to these social questions at some length, Acland disqualifies himself for further discussion and limits his following discussion to "most of what a Physician may venture to remark on the social condition of such a city as Oxford," to wit, "(1) Habitations; (2) Ventilation; (3) Drainage; (4) Medical care of the less affluent classes; (5) The relations between moral and physical well-being" (108)—a broad set of categories indeed and one on which Acland has a great deal left to say, including recommending scientific and religious education for all and recreation in the arts, as "bad music . . . and incorrect drawing" are "as great an intellectual evil as a foul smell is a physical one" (155). Here we see the language associating physical with moral fitness, and moral fitness with culture and the arts, that will recur so frequently in the parliamentary debates of the 1860s on fitness for the franchise, and will be the staples of Ruskin and Matthew Arnold's writings on the relations of culture and citizenship.[9] In a later lecture, Acland is asked to speak on appropriate prints for working people to decorate their homes; he suggests, among other possibilities, geological and physical maps: "Prints for Cottage walls" (7). Category 5 creates a site for Acland to insist on the value of the doctor's professional knowledge to diagnose public issues affecting all classes of society, and implicitly claims an authority equal to that of the clergy who had, up until the 1840s, dominated public conversation about the social meanings of cholera.

Acland also recognizes early on the importance of education for fitness, and connects it repeatedly to public health and sanitation in his *Memoir* on the cholera epidemics in Oxford (1856):

> Upon the judicious Education of the people depends, more than on any other human means, the destiny of our country. God be thanked that each year some ground is gained in the strife against the social evils that sometimes bid fair to overwhelm us. But as long as a large part of our population are, in respect to one or more of the three great portions of their earthly nature, the Physical, Moral and Intellectual, so much lower than they might be, the public opinion, which rules in a constitution such as ours, must be frequently in error. The discussion which is caused by conflict of opinion is nevertheless one of the most efficient means of judicious changes, and of real progress. (142–43)

Physical health is absolutely necessary to the other two categories of development, Acland argues, and, with education, is the primary concern of the medical profession and the state, because finally, "[t]he main object of the State is assuredly to secure, as far as possible, the good conduct of the people" (149)— for which good physical health, and the moral health that depends on it, are prerequisites. As his series of maps moves from the overview of the town to the path of the epidemic on to the home of the individual victim, while simultaneously showing the outward movement of disease from individual to town to region, Acland's text maps the moral and political public sphere onto the physical topography of the individual body to the social body, the sanitary environment to the moral and political one, so that the term he carefully brackets as having assumed—"Civilized Community"—comes to be precisely what is at stake.

The narrative of progress, which is toward a "civilized" state, depends equally on the improvement of the environment and the establishment of a public sphere, both of which depend on, as we have seen in the maps and illustrations, the responsible individual and the home. The domain of the social and "social evils" is precisely where these concerns collide, and wherein the state must intervene to promote the "good conduct" and political fitness of its people, lest the community itself become (or remain) "barbarous." In mapping the sanitary condition, Acland feels he has mapped the social condition; in tracing the progress and failure of sanitary amendment, he implies, he is doing no less than mapping the progress—or potential decline—of Western civilization.

Thus, in the first half of the century, both medics and nonmedics created sanitary maps, but whereas sanitarians were primarily interested in using their maps to illustrate a particular situation or argument, medics often used them as part of a complex reinforcement of their professionalism and its relationship to the public sphere. Their ability to relate the state of the social body to the individual body and its specifically physical health through a geographic representation of community enabled them to make claims for their ability to publicly prescribe. They positioned themselves as social engineers whose interventions into the health of the bodies of Britons and the built environment around them would enable communities to participate appropriately in the march of progress toward an ever more civilized and cultured nation. A further development, however, was about to take place, one that would cement medics' claims to public importance based specifically on a specialized knowledge which would differentiate them from the lay sanitarian as public servant. Acland, with his sophisticated use of multiple maps as sources and ability to reference several variables and levels of representation, was the forerunner of important theories which would be constructed with reference to his maps, but which would also represent arguments for the first time specifically medical—that is, based on knowledge of the body and disease processes as well as an application of scientific methods to large data sets. One of those theories, later memorialized as the medically corrrect one, would a short time later be graphically represented in two key maps by John Snow.

3

Invisible to the Naked Eye

John Snow

Cleanliness . . . and an early application of medicine and medical skill . . . were supposed to be specifics against the contagion. And to a certain extent there is some truth in these views; and it is thus that God enforces on us, by his great and invariable laws of health, the necessity of attention to these sanitary measures. But, pushing that truth too far, men began to map out the geographical boundaries of the malady. . . . Then the selfishness of our nature, leaving the poor in their disease or in their danger to pay the penalty of their localities, was heard to congratulate itself on the comparative safety of its better situations. . . . And then it was . . . that the cholera at one leap passed from the squalid abodes of poverty into the houses which were rejoicing in their comforts, and the streets which were high and clean.

> —Rev. Henry Venn Elliott, "Two Sermons on the Hundred and First and Sixty-Second Psalms as Applicable to the Harvest, the Cholera, and the War"

SNOW AND THE MEDICAL MODEL

PHYSICIAN BENJAMIN WARD RICHARDSON, describing public reaction to the St. James epidemic, remarks, "[S]uch a panic possibly never existed in London since the days of the great plague. People fled from their homes as from instant death, leaving behind them, in their haste, all that they valued most" (xxvi). John Snow's analysis of this epidemic and recommendation to remove the Broad Street pump handle are always prominently featured in medical histories of the period. Histories of medical maps hold up Snow's map of the Broad Street epidemic as the most important development in medical mapping of its era. Despite the dominant sanitary paradigm, Snow positioned himself against the sanitarians. In 1855, he gave evidence before the Select Committee, expressing his conviction that "he was no defender of nuisances, but . . . a bad smell cannot, simply because it is a bad smell, give rise to a specific disease" and that specific diseases were the result of specific disease agents (Richardson xxix).

Snow's famous second edition of *On the Mode of Communication of Cholera* begins with an argument for human transmission of the disease and a history of its movement across Asia and Europe from the Ganges. A substantial portion tracing epidemics in several other areas of London and the United Kingdom generally consists of verbal mapping, with place names and dates, but does not include cartographic representation. The first map is of the St. James outbreak (see fig. 3.1). This is of course the primary topic of the paper and the most impressive to the public not only because of the concentration of deaths there, but because of the fame of the parish as the location of court and metonym for aristocratic wealth of the metropolis, as we will see in chapter 4. Interestingly, it contains no dates, although using dates to show spread was a widespread practice in epidemic mapping. (Snow includes dates and numbers of deaths in a separate table.) Snow states that most deaths took place very close to the pump, but then mentions some which took place further away, in consequence of exposure to the pump water, or those deaths which resulted from exposure in Broad Street, but took place in the country as a result of householders fleeing the city. Snow does not choose to show a larger map with lines connecting such victims to Broad Street, which would provide more complete evidence but lessen the visual impact of the map. He defines the "cholera field" in the following way:

> The dotted line on the map surrounds the sub-districts of Golden Square, St. James's, and Berwick Street, St James's, together with the adjoining portion of the subdistrict of St. Anne, Soho, extending from Wardour Street to Dean St., and a small part of the sub-district of St James's Square enclosed by Marylebone Street, Titchfield Street, Great Windmill Street and Brewer Street. All the deaths from cholera which were registered in the six weeks from 19th August to 30th September within this locality, as well as those persons removed into Middlesex Hospital, are shown in the map by a black line in the situation of the house in which it occurred or in which the fatal attack was contracted. (46)

Additionally, Snow shows the locations of all pumps and adds explanations for why some pumps were less used than others, and why some deaths

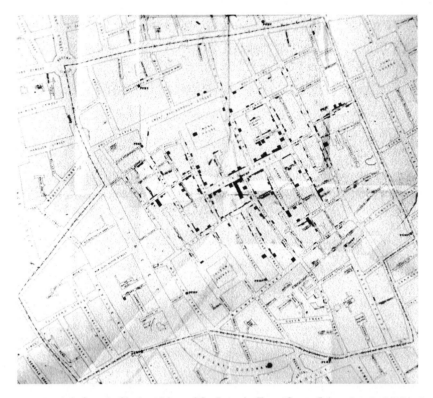

FIGURE 3.1. Snow's Cholera Map of St. James's. From Snow, John. *On the Mode of Communication of Cholera*. 2nd ed., much enlarged. London: John Churchill, 1855.

apparently far from the Broad Street pump are actually related to it. All in all, the map requires a good deal of supplementary verbal explanation, totaling four pages just for the basic clarification of what the reader is looking at. For example, the map aims to show by the locations of the pumps that the Broad Street pump is the culprit. Yet in some heavily visited areas, other pumps are closer. This fact necessitates the explanation that "the water of the pump in Marlborough Street [. . .] was so impure that many people avoided using it," the Rupert Street pump is hard to get to, and the other scattered deaths were all somehow contracted when the victims were closer to the Broad Street pump (*On the Mode* 46–47).

In short, even though Snow was right, there is nothing obvious about the way the map works or the choices Snow made, and in earlier papers on the topic, Snow did not bother to use maps. Yet, for all that, it is, as generations of historians have felt it to be, a striking map. Folding out of the report at a scale of thirty inches to the mile, the map marks death houses with coffin shaped black bars. Where there are several, the results, in a simple black and white line map, are eye catching. And certainly there is a grouping around the Broad Street pump. Still, had a map reader been motivated to find fault, there would be plenty here to undercut Snow's thesis—it is in the text that the objections the map might raise are nullified. It is too often forgotten that this argument was initially widely refuted—by the investigators reporting to the Privy Council, for example—and that Snow did not use the map to convince the guardians to remove the pump handle, but created it long after the fact. Nor did he use it to discover the relationship between water and cholera, a theory he had been working on for some time and had already published in 1849.

What the map does do, and what all disease maps of this period do to some extent, is to redefine a space, usually an urban space, by the relationship of a certain human experience—vulnerability to disease—in relation to some hidden or at least nonobvious feature of the landscape. In this way, maps were very like anatomy "atlases" or pathology texts—they laid bare the invisible relationships between seemingly different things that only the doctor/scientists gaze could discern. In Snow's case, it was water and its flow and the human activities around water that defined a "field" or disease community. The community is demarcated by what we might phrase as the "furthest reach of the disease within a convenient representational area"—in other words, it does not include the cases in the country or in hospitals in another parish. Snow is concerned with origin, and the map is created to argue for that origin. Further, it does not extend to other communities in London that suffered in the 1854–1855 epidemic. Snow maps only the deaths he feels he can trace to the pump. This is essential for his argument, and may also rhetorically play to the perceptions of the residents who, as we shall see, distinguished their epidemic from that of the rabble elsewhere, though Snow pays extensive attention to other areas of London in his text. Unlike many sanitary maps, wherein communities were defined instrumentally by boundaries of parish authority, Snow's map of the St. James's epidemic spills considerably over into St. Anne's Soho. Parish boundaries become less important than the itineraries—the "practice of space"—that link the residents of an area in their use of a common water source. In turn, the anachronic nature of the map freezes that human activity and figures it as a passive spatial relationship.

The next portion of the report doubles back to 1832 as Snow draws larger connections between water quality and disease. He uses tables to show parish variations in mortality and connect them to water supply, first in 1832 and then in 1849 (which also correlates to house values): "A glance at the table shows that in every district to which the supply of Southwark and Vauxhall, or the Lambeth Water Company extends, the cholera was more fatal than in any other district whatever" (*On the Mode* 64). He continues this examination through the most recent epidemic, using more than fourteen tables, mostly from William Farr's evidence, to illustrate various points about population, water purity, season, and so forth.

These tables are extensively discussed, and are themselves far more telling than the map which illustrates them and which Snow does not discuss at all. The map is quite beautiful, though, in three flat colors printed over a black and white map of Southwest London from west to east including Putney to the Isle of Dogs to the north, and to the south of the Thames covering Wimbledon on the west to Sydenham on the east (see fig. 3.2). The colors include red or pink for areas served by the Lambeth Water Company, blue for Southwark and Vauxhall, and purple where the pipes are mingled. The map, obviously a regular commercial map which he has had printed over, contains a good deal of extraneous information (railway lines and such). It shows deaths with small square or rectangular spots, and makes no attempt to correlate

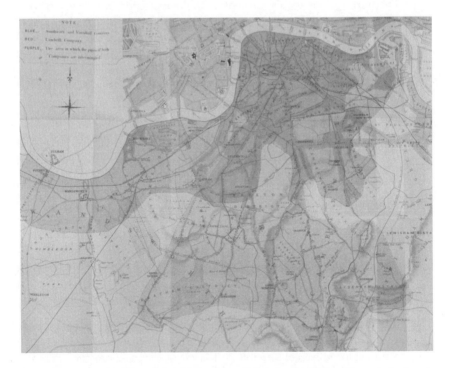

FIGURE 3.2. Snow's Water Map. From Snow, John. *On the Mode of Communication of Cholera.* 2nd ed., much enlarged. London: John Churchill, 1855.

them to structures such as pumps and so forth. This map is much less frequently mentioned by cartographic historians than the Broad Street map.

However, the second map is rhetorically interesting, and was fascinating to its contemporary audience, in that it shows an even less obviously visible relationship between disease and population than the first, more local map. Although Snow's maps were not important in discovering the causal relationships they illustrate, they were certainly important in allowing readers— guided by the expert testimony in the text—to conceptualize such relationships in a new way, having to do with the actions of humans in relation to the environment. Despite the startling argument which it illustrated, the map had the virtue of a certain familiarity—because sanitary theories determined moist areas to be miasmatic, the riverbanks had long been viewed with suspicion— so that there was already a context for understanding the Thames as a threat. Judging from the strong response to this paper, after earlier papers by Snow arguing the same theory had gone unanswered, and judging from the universal use of maps in those reports either attempting to support or refute Snow, the maps had a strong suasive impact.

The water company map does offer a new definition of a human community, much like the Broad Street map, a definition based on multiple factors—location relative to the Thames, to particular piping, and so on, but, perhaps most importantly, as a group of consumers. United both by their access to a geographical resource and by their consumption of a certain consumer good, this community achieves a certain political and legal status through this definition. (The 1867 epidemic sparked parliamentary investigations into the water companies and epidemiological analyses of their product and its sources.) And of course, it also shows the connectedness of a large and widely dispersed group of people through their interactions with the environment. All of these allow different ways of imagining community, and encourage them—by grounding the stakes in something as fundamental as the body and survival itself. Perhaps most importantly, as we saw in chapter 2, medical maps provided doctors with a way to talk about populations in a way legitimated by that medical vision Foucault so compellingly described in *Birth of the Clinic*. Early on, sanitarians and public health legislators slighted doctors, in part because the doctor was perceived to have to do only with individuals and their treatment—inevitably a private affair. Epidemics, for doctors, it was thought, were just large numbers of individual cases. Medical mapping allowed doctors to talk about populations, not in the borrowed terms of sanitarians, who were concerned with what the untrained eye could easily see (or the nose could smell), but in terms uniquely their own, showing relationships not readily visible to the lay observer. It provided doctors with a way of staking out public health as a medical rather than simply a management issue.

John Snow represents a new kind of medical mapmaker, one who departed decisively from the sanitary model of miasmatic spread, and who used maps to advance a more subtle argument, based on a more clearly medical understanding of the body—that is, an understanding of the body based on beliefs about causation which were derived from a surgical model, allowing for specific disease agents. In researching his theory about the waterborne nature of the cholera, Snow himself examined many maps. Snow's several papers before the Broad Street outbreak, arguing the same theory, that is fecal-oral communication especially through contaminated water, referred to maps and reports published elsewhere, and an extensive correspondence with local medics in other cities, although, as I have said, these papers were not illustrated with maps of their own. He refers especially to the literature surrounding cholera in India. In 1849 for example, he speaks of his conviction of human carriage derived from the Indian literature from 1817 onward (5), and argues for the fecal-oral route, noting, "Many of the patients attributed their illness to the water" which smelled bad (Snow, *On the Mode* 8–9). He also was careful to examine all the available maps on the cholera in England, including Shapter's. Like Acland, he was interested in tracing an historical and geographical relationship which required the comparison of multiple documents, although, unlike Acland, his argument is not best served by encoding that longer history in the map, as he wishes to draw attention to the geography of a very particular epidemic.

Although Shapter does not show pump locations, the proximity of the concentration of deaths, and especially earlier deaths, near the river in Shapter's map may have been useful to Snow—although the population is also concentrated in that same area, making the map a good candidate to support either sanitarian arguments against crowding or statistical arguments about proportional per capita distribution. Shapter does include a great deal of information in his text about the locations and availability of water sources as part of his sanitary argument. Snow corresponded with Shapter, and refers to maps of sewer locations with which Shapter provided him (Snow, *On the Mode* 98). He observes that Shapter mentions that in 1832, most town dwellers used river water whereas in the following epidemic, the town was well sewered and well supplied with water, and only twenty died there, the victims mostly having come from elsewhere. By the third epidemic, only one death took place in Exeter. Snow also refers to studying a map of Hull, "furnished me in 1849 by Dr. Horner of Hull" (*On the Mode* 101). He often mentions other works which we know contained maps, even if he does not refer specifically to the maps themselves; he mentions consulting various local sanitary reports, for example on Birmingham, most of which were supplemented with maps *(On the Mode)*, as this practice of including them in local sanitary reports became widespread from the late 1840s on. In short, Snow was working within a context of a genre defined in part by the sanitary map and his discussion shows that he is using these maps as a research tool to support and supplement his own analysis.

What Snow does not show is as important as what he does. He does not show dates, lines of spread, the locations of nuisances, drains, or sewers, as many before him had done. He also does not show geological features such as elevation or soil type, which he could certainly have done on the second map, although he mentions with interest the work of the American John Lea, who had attempted such a correlation. He ignores all of these common devices because they are not germane to the argument he wants to make—as we shall see, a response to his argument is the General Board Report, which does display some of these sanitary features. In the light of such comments as Robinson's—"Although Snow did not know what caused the cholera, the structure of the distribution of deaths as revealed by the mapping convinced him that water from a particular well was the local source" (*Early Thematic Mapping* 172–73)—it is important to remind ourselves that Snow's map worked as well as it did because it was a highly selective illustration of a hypothesis, not a research tool in the first instance: he had worked out his theory well in advance of the creation of this map.[1] But the rhetoric of this map is based on the truth claims of cartography in this period, and it is quite possible that the map came to seem less and less refutable, less and less an argument and more a representation of reality, as it became detached from the immediate context of 1855. What is important here is that for the first time, the map is clearly and consciously used to advance an argument, not with a belief that the map will transparently show the truth, but with the conviction that the truth is more persuasive represented cartographically than otherwise, and the rhetoric of the map is carefully controlled to heighten the effect of Snow's argument.

These maps offer little sense of lived space, a task which is taken up by their accompanying narrative. Shapter and Snow, for example, both provide ample explanation of why people used one water source rather than another, and how apparently anomalous deaths were to be reconciled with the existing narrative. This provides something of the sense of perceived and lived space the map lacks. We learn of the practices and preferences of the people within that environment: how the brewers were untouched because they drank only beer, how one lady sent her servants well out of their way because she preferred the taste of the pump at Broad Street. But visual representations of data tended toward abstraction and homogenization, organizing their reader-cueing strategies by assigning equivalent values to apparently equivalent spaces and simplifying out data that complicated those representations.

In this same period, we see the increasing homogenization of verbal case studies and the introduction of standardized charts which simplified the collection and analysis of data, but tended also to structure the encounter of the patient and healthcare worker in terms of general norms rather than individual experiences. Although both patients' case charts and maps emerge from the increasing importance of statistics and the Euclidean vision they depend on, it is probably not too much to hypothesize that the spatialization of individual experience in a chart may have been facilitated by a medical and social imaginary nurtured on the more intuitive visual representation of geographical space and connection of individual bodies' health to that spatialized visual display. The details of lived experience and personal character that would have been so important to diagnosis a few decades earlier are now relegated to the status of secondary information. They come into the narrative primarily to explain the incursion of lived space's irrationality, which the map's implicit reliance on conceived space makes it incapable of representing—for example, the map's use of proximity to the well to mark the well's dangerousness fails confronted with some individuals' apparently irrational use of a well which is not the closest one to them. Narrative becomes a vehicle for the explanation of individual abnormality; the norm can be represented visually.

In short, although cholera maps of the time actually tell or prove very little without the accompanying text, the mere existence of the map itself could have a powerful legitimating effect. As we saw earlier, maps evoked potent claims to transparency and truth—even when the truth had to be carefully defined verbally to be visible. And, increasingly in this period, social truths were that which could be represented primarily visually, giving narrative the role of supplementing and explaining that truth.[2] And those who refuted Snow had to have recourse to the medium of the map to do so.

Several responses were published. The Royal College of Physicians, represented by Baly and Gull, considered Snow's theory and rejected it in their detailed analysis of the epidemic. However, their report was drawn up, apparently, before Snow's 1855 map was in print. The General Board of Health published what was probably the weightiest early response to the outbreak—and to Snow (General Board of Health, Medical Council). Their report reveals a complex local dialogue on the etiology of the disease, in which local residents drew on local history and maps and urban legend to respond to the outbreak and also to sanitary improvements which had been underway at the time of the epidemic, as well as internecine battles between medical researchers:

> We found two opinions, amongst others, prevalent throughout the neighbourhood; one, that the disturbance of the old burying ground was the chief cause of the outbreak of Cholera, the ravages of which, many of the inhabitants maintained, followed the line of the new sewer, the other, that a pump in Broad Street was at the bottom of the mischief. Neither of these causes, we believe, affords a satisfactory reason for the outbreak; both, we suspect, have been prominently put forth by interested persons, who were desirous of

diverting the current of popular indignation from their own particular nuisances. For example, we found the owner of the monster slaughter-house in
Marshall Street, and who also has an interest in the tripe-boiling establishment adjoining, to be one of the loudest and most eager in declaiming
against the sewers . . . [but this is not borne out]. . . . As to [the pump] . . .
we are bound to say that there are some cases of disease and death which we
find ourselves unable to explain upon any other hypothesis. (Fraser, Hughes,
and Ludlow 150–153)

"The old burying ground" referred to a plague pit on the estate grounds on
which St. James's rested—the burial ground dating back, then, to the sixteenth
century. The notion that it was directly under Broad Street was based on the
Commissioners of Sewers' map, a map subsequently revised by comparison to
a supposedly more accurate map from the Craven estate which showed the
true location of the burial ground at some distance from that spot. The author
lumps in the supporters of Snow's theory with "interested persons" like the
slaughterhouse owner, yet, finally, must admit that there are deaths that cannot be accounted for in other ways. A "corrected" map attached elsewhere in
the report is not specifically referred to but reflects this narrative (see fig. 3.3).
The map is responsive to Snow's argument and to the other rumors, showing
the old sewers, the new sewer, the location of the Lord Craven estate and the
"erroneous" location of the plague pit shown in the map of the Commissioners of Sewers—which indicates that someone had gone early on to look at the
Commissioner of Sewers' map in order to support the plague pit claim. The
spot map is detailed, at eighty-eight feet to one inch, and shows all deaths by
small rectangles, with differently oriented rectangles to show whether the victim was a resident of the area or not. They also mark pumps, side entrances,
ventilators, and sewer grates, distinguishing between trapped and untrapped.
    Snow's pamphlet was finished on December 11, 1854, and published in
1855 *(On the Mode)*. He refers to Scot's 1824 report, Baly, of Baly and Gull's
Royal College of Physicians Report (1854), and several reports from local sanitary authorities and from India (with maps). It seems likely that Snow's map
was completed before the General Board's. It is likely that the authors of the
board's report would have seen Snow's map before it went to press in any case,
as Snow had been courteously helped with access to all information on cholera
mortality at the General Registrar's Office as it came in. The General Board's
map, constructed by Fraser, Ludlow, and Hughes, follows the basic plan of
Snow's, though it is larger and shows more detail, including house numbers.
It also covers somewhat less area, not going much east of Regent Street,
whereas Snow includes material to Bond Street on the southeast portion of
the map. The General Board uses the Commissioners of Sewers' map and
updates it by consulting the Craven estate archives to show a "more accurate"
location of the plague pit. Snow also includes a great deal of material outside

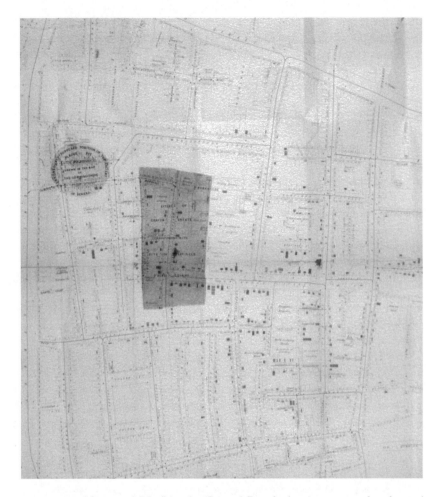

FIGURE 3.3. "Corrected Map" by the General Board, showing supposed and actual location of plague pit: detail. From General Board of Health. Medical Council. *Appendix to Report of the Committee for Scientific Inquiries in Relation to the Cholera Epidemic of 1854.* London: Eyre and Spottiswoode, 1855.

of the epidemic area, but only maps deaths within the lines, which gives the visual impression of much more concentration, whereas the board includes no area outside of the boundaries of their area of investigation. Pumps are drawn as smaller dots on the board's map, while sewer symbols compete for attention with the markers of deaths. The board's report shows more deaths, interestingly. For example, on Poland Street, Snow shows three deaths at a location where the board shows four: two residents and two nonresidents. The board also shows the locations of cow sheds and so on to bolster a sanitary argument.

Despite the fact that this is as often called the Golden Square outbreak as the Broad Street outbreak, there were very few deaths anywhere near Golden Square, and the Golden Square registration district suffered proportionately with the adjacent Berwick Street registration district. Snow does map two deaths right across the street from Golden Square, but in the greater detail of the board map—three times the size of the Snow map—we see one death there, oriented toward upper John Street (that is around the corner from rather than facing Golden Square), and that is within a building marked "Homeopathic Hospital." The impact of the many deaths at 38 Broad Street on Snow's map is somewhat lessened by seeing on the board map that this is a factory employing many hands and not a private house. However, finally it is clear in both maps that Broad Street and areas surrounding its intersection with Cambridge Street and Little Windmill Street are clearly the epicenter of the outbreak. Despite the board's concession that the pump was clearly somehow involved, however, the report finally concludes in favor of a sanitarian argument, referring to the upcoming debate on a bill which they hope will consolidate power of sanitary authorities and give them power to act. It was, perhaps, not the best time to advance an argument which might appear to detract from the sanitary model.

In the same report, Robert Dundas Thomson attempts to refute both Snow's theory and his opponents under the existing elevation theory of William Farr, a theory which connected low elevation with mortality, and was consistent with the "heavier air" concept of miasma:

> The Facts connected with the occurrence of cholera on river margins have been elaborately urged by Dr. Snow in favour of the Indian theory, while the same circumstances have been most ingeniously applied by another theorist to the use of autumnal stores of unsound flour. The law of elevation, however, established by Dr. Farr, takes cognizance of such facts and affords a general view of the subject. (R. D. Thomson 185)

What is interesting here is that both Snow and his unknown opponent are attempting to explain the epidemic according to an interrelationship of environment and behaviors, whereas Farr reads the disease as the results of geographic laws on passive human bodies. However, all three seek a primarily spatial explanation for the epidemic.

This spatialization of epidemiological research in Britain was not now restricted to the surface topography of land and built environment, but already assumed a palimpsestic historical organization of space which we have seen in the local inhabitants' recourse to maps of the old plague burial ground and in Acland's map of the same period. Seeking an explanation in history and the historical uses of space, residents of St. James's use a geological model that assumes that strata of the ground under their feet contain both evidence and potentially active residue of past uses of the environment. The appendix, however, also has recourse to a model of a palimpsest of microspaces within macrospaces, containing a street-by-street and house-by-house mapping of the microorganisms found in the water of every place where cholera occurred (with hand colored pictures) and narratives (by Hassall). Attentive to Snow's theory, the report also summarizes microorganic content by water company. The enclosed map (fig. 3.3, described above) of the St. James's epidemic is accompanied by charts which map the houses in order, so that the report maps space at the level of the community, the historical use of the land during an earlier epidemic (the plague), the microlevel, and the structural level of individual houses—a mapping which mediates between several conceptions of meaningful space, from that of legal units of property and historical use of terrain to the more slippery one of water content (see fig. 3.4).

The mapping of water flora and fauna, of course, captures only the ephemeral presence of particular organisms at a particular time in a single droplet, yet it implies a tentative belief in a constant presence of harmful or harmless organisms in a particular location; the attribution of different flora to different water companies poses a more trenchant critique. Snow's appeal to a narrative of progress and melioration is opposed by a complex counternarrative, one also conscious of an appeal to progress but simultaneously suspicious of it—what if laying down the new sewers is not an improvement over the past, but instead invokes that past? The past is contained in the present land, like the fossils which were then unsettling traditional views of the earth's age—still dangerous, still active, that past can erupt into the present, the plague unleashed through misguided attempts at improvement. This narrative of an eternally present threat of return—a mythic, cyclical narrative of monumental time as opposed to historical time—is the dark underside of the linear narrative of progress which both sanitary and medical science offered.

Sharon Marcus identifies the legend of the haunted London lodging house as a particularly mid-nineteenth-century narrative: "[G]hosts represented a drag on modernity, an exception in a regime defined by new technologies of visualization and surveillance designed to abolish all hidden dangers, including specters" (117), and here we see something of the same gesture in the notion of an underground haunted by a barbaric disease out of the distant past.[3] The urban space conceived by social practitioners was a forward looking one—thoroughly modern and anticipating the modernist, it was envisioned in opposition to a past which seemed aligned with barbarism and which marked the city from below, complicating its potential transparency and cleanliness. The valuable part of the past was its monumentality, its evocation of national history, but its dark side was the material trace of barbarity

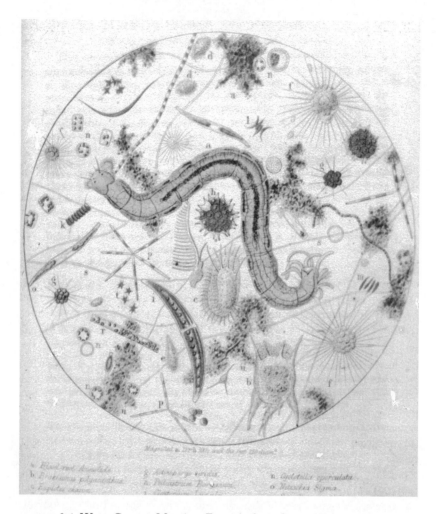

FIGURE 3.4. Water Content Mapping, Example from General Board *Report:* detail. From General Board of Health. Medical Council. *Appendix to Report of the Committee for Scientific Inquiries in Relation to the Cholera Epidemic of 1854.* London: Eyre and Spottiswoode, 1855.

within the structure of the city itself. The perceived space of the city was marked by this ambivalence—pride in its historic identity as metropole, and fascinated fear of its historic reputation as site of disease, plague, and crime.

Snow found an ally in Henry Whitehead, the curate of St. Luke's, Berwick, who would later be asked to join the vestry committee and would publish an arduously researched corroboration of Snow's theory. He wrote his own pamphlet on the epidemic, *The Cholera in Berwick Street*, in 1854. The pamphlet begins with a map of the parish as a frontispiece, and he begins his article with a verbal mapping which he enhances by a diagram published in the margin: "If a person were to start travelling from the western end of Broad Street . . . and [walk along a specified route], he would pass . . . forty-five houses, of which only six escaped without a death" (1). Not having satisfied himself with a catalogue of streets, he continues, "[A]n easy way suggests itself to his [the author's] mind by which he may enable anyone to ascertain for himself, almost by a glance at a map of London, the streets and parts of streets throughout which the disease may be said to have performed literally a *house to house visitation*," and he commences to describe an irregular triangle comprising a number of streets, which he also has printed, set into the left margin of the page and displacing the print around it (2, emphasis in original).

Whitehead uses his clerical relationship with the residents to recheck Snow's information, beginning by eliciting details of residents' practices of the region in this triangular area. Unlike Snow's vision, which begins with an abstract sense of the area defined by the outbreak and then focuses in more narrowly to identify individual deaths and illnesses, Whitehead's is a clergyman's vision—one based on intimate knowledge of the area and the residents—which begins at the level of the street and the telling metaphor of "house to house visitation." This was a method beloved of sanitary inspectors—Fraser, Hughes, and Ludlow of the general board visit eight hundred houses in their follow-up to Snow's article—but also of philanthropic visitors of all kinds. Only after that peripatetic mapping does Whitehead imagine the bird's-eye view inherent in a cartogram as the most effective way to communicate with readers who do not know the area, to make visible at a glance the larger relations of deaths to spatial location. Whitehead presents himself as originally skeptical of Snow, having been won over by painstaking correlation of Snow's data; this evidently repositions Whitehead spatially as well, causing him to envision the area scientifically, as an abstract mapping of mortality, as well as a series of well-known streets, houses, and individuals.

Whitehead was apparently invited to participate in the parish's independent report to the vestry by the Cholera Inquiry Committee (St. James, Westminster) along with the original committee itself, Snow, and other interested parties, and the pamphlet described above derives from his report, which was submitted May 8, 1855. Mr. York, an engineer who investigated the sewer next to the pump in Broad Street, submitted a separate report with a diagram of the area under Broad Street, finding communication between cesspit and pump on May 1, 1855, and thus confirming the potential for contamination of the well by the infant identified as the vector (see fig. 3.5). The cutaway view of a house and the area beneath it is not new—

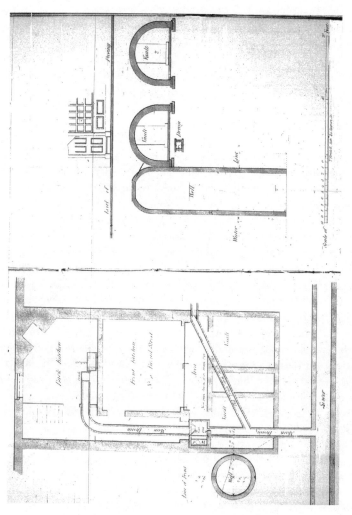

FIGURE 3.5. Well Diagram in General Board Report. From General Board of Health. Medical Council. *Appendix to Report of the Committee for Scientific Inquiries in Relation to the Cholera Epidemic of 1854.* London: Eyre and Spottiswoode, 1855.

many sanitary illustrations drew cross sections of buildings, showing the cellars or sewers below—but these earlier illustrations were fanciful illustrations of general truths (Gavin's lodging house) rather than scientific documents of specific conditions.

The combination of Snow's mapping and Mr. York's drawing of the proximity of the well and cesspit revealed hidden features of the built environment which were dangerous to health and which could only be revealed by experts, medical or structural. Whitehead could verify Snow's thesis with his house-to-house data checking, but neither he nor any other layperson would have developed Snow's hypothesis, an educated guess, indeed, based on a detailed professional knowledge, not only of the body and theories of its functioning, but of earlier professional publications on the cholera. Whitehead carefully notes his relationship to the limitations of the different kinds of knowledge:

> The subject of defective drainage ought perhaps not to be handled by any but practical men. As there is little need however of a special or technical education to render one sensible of greviously offensive stench, I may at least venture upon the assertion that many of the house drains in Broad St. are in a condition peremptorily demanding the attention of gentlemen professionally acquainted with such matters. (in *Report on the Cholera Outbreak in the parish of St. James's*, 151)

A decade earlier, of course, under Chadwick, there would have been no need to defend the validity, and in fact, priority of such common sense perceptions. Snow's report inaugurated a new era and new standard of evidence or, more accurately, introduced the public to the emerging standards of the medical professional with surgical training in morbid anatomy and tissue theory.

The *Report on the Cholera Outbreak in the Parish of St. James's* compiled by the vestry committee contains a map, explained on the frontispage:

> This Map is the same as that which illustrated the Report of Messrs. Fraser, Ludlow and Hughes [that is, in the general board report's appendix to the report to the general board] on the Cholera outbreak in this district. It is founded on the Map published in Mr. Cooper's Report to the Commissioners of Sewers; but St. Anne's Court and the neighbourhood have been added to it, and the fatal attack which occurred in the district throughout the whole epidemic have been inserted in their respective localities where they could be accurately determined.

In the text, the authors note that the Commissioners of Sewers' map was created in response to their investigation of the epidemic in September 1854; the vestry also consults the Craven estate archives. The map is reproduced faithfully and then given two additions: 1851 sewers are picked out in pale blue and the recent sewer additions are colored pale pink. But most tellingly, in a report which is completely sympathetic to Snow's argument, a circle has been drawn with a compass around the "cholera field" in which the Broad Street pump is the center. Even though this, as a St. James's parish report, actually leaves outside the circle St. Anne's Court (Soho), which was hard hit and which Snow included in his map, it is mutely eloquent, and dramatizes the clustering of deaths around the pump, making them appear even more evenly distributed than they are (see fig. 3.6). The text notes, "It was only in a singularly well-defined portion of [the districts] that the influence of the *great* outbreak was felt. . . . Reference to the map . . . will render this description easily understood" (16).

Clearly, the vestry is sympathetic to Snow, and one might speculate that may have had something to do with the refutation of the stigma and implied social irresponsibility attributable to a parish suffering from a filth disease. However, a more charitable view might have it that, as the vestry is most aware of the habits of the local population, they are in a better position to be persuaded by the truth of Snow's science than the board, which had itself a vested interest in the sanitary idea. In any case, there were clearly felt to be sides to be taken in the dispute. We see in the vestry report the desire to reinforce Snow's claim, and that this involves not only the careful construction of a map which both recapitulates Snow's findings and responds to local lay hypotheses about etiology (the plague pit), but also the legitimation of an engineer's report surveying the condition of the well and cesspool and the additional legitimation of the clergy's point of view—at the same time that the clergyman acknowledges that his own credentials to discourse authoritatively about the state of piping and of medical subjects are already, perhaps fatally, undermined as not "practical." The board, in response, feels the necessity of a detailed chemical and microscopic examination of both water and air, responding to Snow's mapping of space with its own multilayered mapping also based on a specifically scientific knowledge. The days of easy appeal to smell and sight are over, though the sanitary explanation will persist as a viable argument in these overtly scientific writings.

Several significant effects on the course of medical mapping are traceable to this moment and the flurry of responses surrounding Snow. Most crucial is that most English maps would now routinely follow multiple variables, and would rarely be produced de novo, but would refer to a history, not only of data (mortality, weather conditions) but of medical cartography. Another important result was that water supply would now be always included as an important category of scrutiny; the Thames, especially, would now be permanently and distrustfully referenced as both the unifying feature of the London landscape and a source of the city's mortality, its characteristic filth and disease. Although the Thames's pollution was already well known under the san-

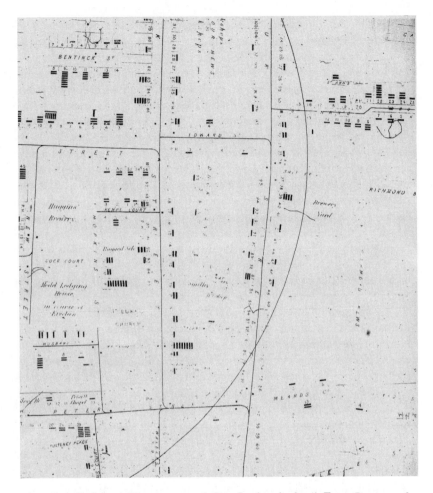

FIGURE 3.6. St. James's Vestry map, excluding St. Anne's: detail. From *Report on the Cholera Outbreak in the Parish of St. James's, Westminster, During the Autumn of 1854.* Presented to the Vestry by the Cholera Inquiry Committee, July 1855. London: J. Churchill, 1855.

itarians, it was part of a general campaign against dirt and damp encompassing all waterside areas. Snow's figures could not be ignored, however, even by them, and now it was the drinking of dirty water that came to mind, the invasion of the body by the city's wastes. John Simon, in his General Board of Health report, *Report on the Last Two Cholera Epidemics of London, as Affected by the Consumption of Impure Water,* bases his extended map of the metropolitan water companies on the same scheme as Snow's and admits that the

Southwark and Vauxhall Company's water from Battersea was "the filthiest stuff ever drunk by a civilized community" (5).

The demonization of the Thames, which corresponded well to sanitarians' long-standing observations that the low-lying, damp areas near the river were insalubrious, enabled a certain shorthand. London had always been mapped with the Thames as its most significant geographical, mercantile, and visual feature, and the riverbanks had for many years been associated with miasma and pollution. As early as 1852, the *Report on the Mortality of Cholera in England: 1848–1849* contains an innovative schematic map of London subdistricts, simplifying actual topography in favor of an abstract overview (see fig. 3.7). The Thames is shown as a straight line, and the positions of subdistricts are shown relative to each other in the simplest sense, by placing text about mortality ratios next to each other in rough relationship to the place to which the text refers. Topography disappears in favor of an absolute distinction between north and south of the river, as all parishes south of the river appear at the same level, despite the fact that there is a significant difference in placement. (Of course, this map is intended to be read in relation to the many other maps contained in the report.)

Cartographic historians have said that there is a trend toward increasing sophistication in mapping in this period, which, as I have said earlier, does not bear up under scrutiny. But what cartographic historians interested in topographically realistic maps have missed is the increasing trend in some areas of thematic cartography toward schematization and abstraction, of which this is an excellent example. (One might think today of the London tube map, an excellent intuitive guide to transport, but one that distorts the actual terrain of the city to an unrecognizable extent in the interests of its primary purpose.) The use of abstract maps, which we also saw earlier in Oxford, assumes a reader who can supply the missing information, and also supply a sophisticated reading schema which will sort necessary from unnecessary information, and information based on typical "realist" cartographic protocols (a northeast line still means northeast) from those for which realist demands may be discarded (a line that is twice as long as another may not accurately represent ratios of space). It also—and this is crucial—implies a space susceptible to abstraction. If Britain is a space of palimpsest, implying layers of history-containing spaces which encode different levels of progress in a kind of layered narrative, it is also a space susceptible to perfection, perfection being the reconstruction of space in the image of a more perfect and pellucid abstraction. In the abstract maps, one sees through the irrelevant presence of a certain topography—a hill, a crowded street—to the essential truths of space and spatial relations between essential features. Now attention focused on the actual flow of water and its relation to the city. London could be easily conceived as a totality, a single connected body, relative to its great river.

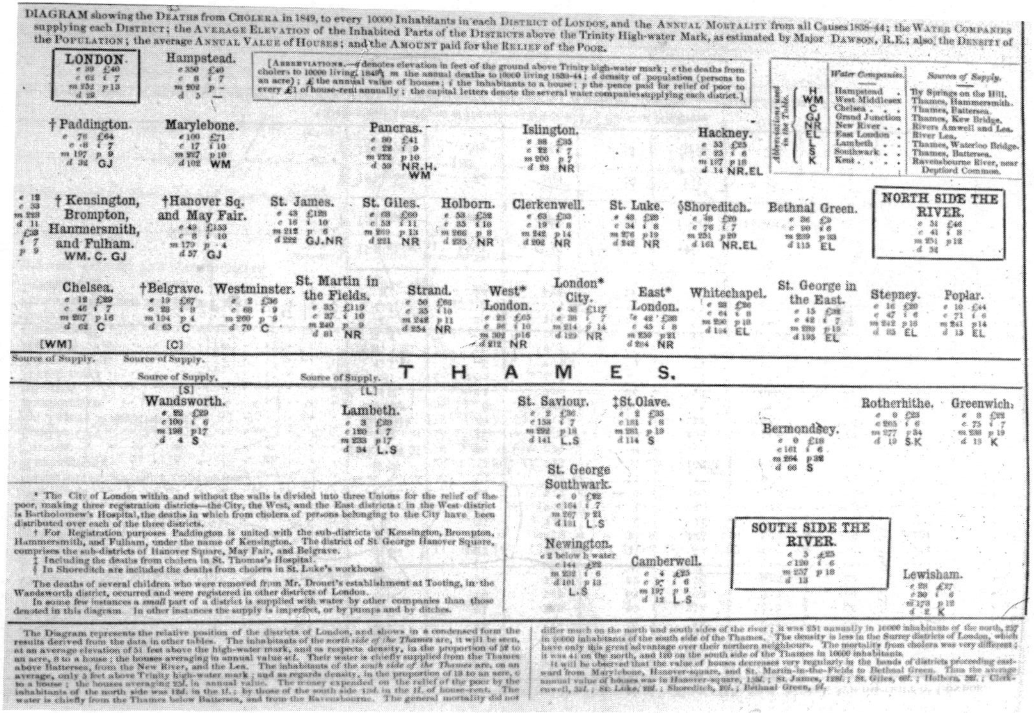

FIGURE 3.7. Schematic Map of London Cholera Mortality. From *Report on the Mortality of Cholera in England: 1848–1849.* London: W. Clowes and Sons, 1852.

Earlier sanitary mapping, under Chadwick, tended to define communities in terms of a responsibility to cleanliness and to controlling the dirty and vicious tendencies of the lower classes—a maternal combination of housekeeping, punishments, and exhortations against bad behavior. The citizen's responsibility was to directly and visually monitor the community, and attempt to redeem the childlike, "barbaric" underclass, presumed directly responsible for lack of cleanliness. With the emergence of the medical model in the late 1850s, however, we see an increasing emphasis on the role of hidden relations that can only be interpreted by medics, surveyors, and engineers. The citizens delegate individual authority to these experts, who then represent that authority and intervene in the physical infrastructure of the urban body in the interest of the community. Social mapping begins to split off—poverty and crime are still in the domain of the interested (and increasingly feminine) individual volunteer who maternally attempts to modify behavior, such as the Bible ladies and Octavia Hills. Sanitary mapping, however, concerns itself with an environment which is seen as deterministically related to disease, even though the choice of living in that environment is still seen as a culpable decision—a perversion of the natural desire for cleanliness. Such maps served to construct a vision of the city and its populations as a totality or organism which could be understood spatially and treated to achieve compliance with an ideal of urban transparency and conformity between geographic factors and human behavior. Abstract mapping reduced the community to its essential (and largely nonhuman) elements and posited a utopian abstract space in which only ideally functional elements had meaning and thus were visible. It posited the possibility of a space with all "noise," all irrelevant and therefore destructive distractions eliminated.

If barbarism is a feature of landscape, often below the surface in its sewerage, its cesspools and wells, its soil quality and the level of the water table, it is a history which can be fixed, purged. Barbarism can also result from the imposition of the perils of modernity on what was formerly a perfectly civilized, but is now an inadequate infrastructure—that is, if the massing of bodies in the modern city is a species of barbarity, improving water supply and sewerage, as well as housing, can create conditions in which civilizing, cleansing, and separating those massed bodies becomes possible. Matching landscape, both natural and built, to properly socialized bodies engaging in properly socialized behaviors is a matter of eliminating these layers of dissonance and reinscribing all within a single layer of time—modernity. However, in order to do this, all those layers must be mapped to identify the points of dissension. Thus we see micromappings of districts—not only street by street, but house by house and finally down to the level of microfauna in some cases. For example, as we have seen, the Broad Street epidemic which proved so fruitful for Snow's investigations provoked many other mappings, including one that mapped the microorganisms present in the water house by house.

Thus the city and its maps function as palimpsests, showing levels of space and discrepancies between times—the time of modernity and the barbaric relics of the past which infect the modern body (largely, though not entirely through the bodies of the backwards, barbaric working classes and Irish underclass). Abstract maps are both a means of achieving a more perfectly modern space and its ideal representation (see Pike). Old Father Thames and his filthy water, representing sewage, the eruption of the grotesque lower bodily strata into the civilized realm of the modern self, become both a problem to be resolved in the name of the modern city and the characteristic sign of the unregenerate city itself.

As we have seen, medical mapping allowed medics to cultivate a unique professional voice in public affairs. It also envisioned (and thus, in part, created) a larger spatial entity as vitally connected and participating in the same structure, as in Snow's water maps of London and those which followed. If one portion of that structure was unhealthy, it could affect the entire organism through its circulatory mechanisms. Unlike, say, Gavin's report, which emphasized the obscurity and isolation of Bethnal Green even while it gestured toward the compromised health of the urban whole, Snow's work vitally connects the visually and imaginatively isolated outbreak in St. James's with the entire urban epidemic, and with portions of the city located far from each other, through its water conduits. The city itself, then, could be seen anatomically as an organism, with circulatory systems vulnerable to contamination which extended throughout the entire urban body rather than miasmatically within a small radius; invisible underground conduits would carry infection even to apparently "clean and sweet" areas—a point reinforced by the irony that most residents drank from the Broad Street pump because the water tasted better than that of surrounding pumps. As Snow pointed out, decaying organic matter actually aerated the water; it was precisely that which made the water dangerous which made it seem most pure to the inexpert senses.

Further, Snow's work located the evil below the surface, within the "body" of the city and requiring a physician's analysis and a quasi-surgical intervention; the city itself came to be seen as a problematic organism, related both to its geography (poor drainage, water sources) and the activity of its population (drinking from particular sources, disposal of waste), which itself was in part determined by geography (people have to have water; they get it where they can). No longer could the city be seen as a basically healthy organism containing some specific problem locations, requiring local cosmetic intervention. The years of attention to morbid anatomy and increasing importance of surgeons as a professional group since the 1830s almost certainly had a part in this shift from surface to depth, as it did in the shift from a sanitary to a medical model, as did the departure of Chadwick and the ascendancy of Farr.

The maps also, in their anatomical rhetoric, treat the city as analogous to a body. This is particularly true of the larger scale maps, such as Snow's second one. The city, a fusion of human bodies and geographic setting, "sickens" with contamination. The human bodies, invisible on the map of homogenous space that is the city, are represented by the personification of the city itself as population. The mapmakers and readers are obsessed with visibility and truth; the idea that the maps will make "visible at a glance" the problems and relationships under study is pervasive. Some such wording almost always accompanies the mapmaking enterprise. After all, the map purports merely to represent what is there—a material reality. Yes at the same time, thematic maps, especially medical ones, attempt to uncover hidden relationships, and as we have seen, often are not clear at all without the doctor's accompanying text. Here too, there is a truth claim: the doctor will make visible the invisible, but the untrained eye will still require a legend to see the reality so clearly on display.

Instead of the individual parishes which middle-class people must care for, as in Gavin's work, we see a large interconnected city wherein disease in one portion threatens the life of all; furthermore, remedies must be applied to the invisible underground structure of the city through its circulatory mechanisms—its sewers and cesspits, its water conduits—rather than the removal of obvious superficial nuisances like dungheaps. The poverty of the dwellers of Golden Square is not seen as an important factor (in fact, Snow deemphasizes the fact that the outbreak is in a slum, concentrating on promoting an image of the neighborhood as habited by respectable artisans, probably in order to discourage recourse to sanitary explanations).[4] Conceiving a geographical construct as a community and in turn as a body enabled these medics and social experts to bring the city conceptually into the domain of the social. One understanding of the city—as a region filled with private properties—was powerful in militating against centralized governmental intervention in sanitation and housing. If the city, however, were not merely a dwelling place of inappropriate bodies, but identical with them, then the city itself entered the legitimate domain of social intervention, which ultimately authorized not only sanitary, educational, and housing programs directed by government, but eventually allowed them to be government supported as well.

Benjamin Ward Richardson supposes that Snow's work did not circulate widely, but certainly Snow was widely respected and published in reputable journals at this point, and had reprinted and circulated many of his works in tract form; he was also widely cited, though he does correspond with various journals to correct others' lack of acknowledgment of his priority.[5] In short, the medical community was certainly aware of Snow's theories fairly early on, even though it took a long while for them to be completely accepted. Significantly, William Farr of the General Registrar's Office took a keen interest in

Snow's work and data, though he initially opposed his conclusions. In the 1860s, Farr himself proclaimed Snow correct (though he had agreed with some of Snow's conclusions as early as 1852), but even then, most doctors did not subscribe to the belief in a specific disease agent, although the interaction of environmental effects and contaminated water were believed to be deleterious. As late as 1867, D. K. Whittaker says that cholera "germs" (here used in the sense of "cause," not the later meaning of a specific unicellular disease agent) are commonly held to be contained in the excreta of cholera sufferers—a theory he attributes to Orton, not Snow—but also says "it is usual to hold that in their recent state they do not propagate the disease, that they have first to go through a process of fermentation"(25), a theory also championed by William Farr. In any case, by the 1860s, Snow is rarely *not* mentioned, and the first map, at least, was widely perused and imitated.

William Farr's *Report on the Cholera Epidemic of 1866 in England* (1868) unreservedly acknowledges Snow to have been correct, referring to Snow's papers extending back to 1849, to the General Board's report of 1855, and to the subsequent committee report by Snow, Whitehead et al. published in 1855 (St. James). The whole report is geared toward examining the condition of the water, and two choropleth maps show mortality and correlate with water supply. The water companies came under public investigation for their role in providing unsafe water in the 1866 epidemic. (Their claims to have provided only filtered water became laughable in the face of consumers' evidence that live eels had emerged from some pumps [*Appendix to Report From Select Committees on East London Water Bills*, 355–57]). The water companies' desperate counter that the liveliness of the eels proved the salubrity of the water was not persuasive.)[6] By this time, maps had become the unquestioned and privileged tool for epidemiological study, and indeed, for all statistical research on the social body. Farr writes, with some satisfaction, that, "personal inspection, the use of maps, such information as we had the means of getting from the registrars, the health officers and other persons, enabled us week by week to track the epidemic through this vast metropolis" (*Report on the Cholera* 98)[7]—a metropolis at last, for a select few, visible at a glance.

PART III

Narrating Metropolitan Space

4

A Tale of Two Parishes

Place and Narrative in the
London Cholera Epidemic of 1854

Of course, in London, he met with every variety of contrast. On the one hand riches and plenty, and on the other poverty and starvation . . . were all found side by side wherever you wandered through that great city; and he could not better illustrate the contrast than by quoting a song he once purchased of a street singer. . . . [T]he song was entitled "St. James and St. Giles." . . .

"In St. James there's one Palace I swear;
In St. Giles, Gin Palaces everywhere;
In St. James, Pall Mall is considered polite;
In St. Giles Pell Mell in the gutter they fight;
In St. James they lie down on pillows by score;
In St. Giles the same, but it's down on the floor."

Such was the style of the song, and it was a fair representation of the moral and social contrasts presented by the two great neighboring parishes.

—George Wilson M'Cree, "Day and Night in St. Giles:
A Lecture Delivered in the British Schoole Room,
Bishop Auckland on Tuesday, June 17th, 1862"

WE HAVE SEEN SOMETHING of how Snow's views were argued and contested in relation to sanitary and medical conceptions of space. But of course, these conceptions themselves did not operate in a vacuum. Snow's arguments were consumed within a context of multiple perceptions and lived experiences of space, both by local residents of the area and others. This chapter will seek to recover some of those other perceptions and narratives, to which Snow's conception of space had to address itself and against which it was evaluated. The location of the epidemic in a space of singular importance in the London imaginary had much to do with Snow's reception; it also leaves us with a uniquely well-documented response to the challenge posed by medical mapping. This chapter explores, through one example, the context of reception of medical maps: the existing narratives and readings of the city's spaces, the myths that circulated about these spaces and their inhabitants, and, to some extent, the lived experience of these spaces that informed these perceptions.

Within narratives of social life, place occupies a peculiar position, as both itself the subject of narratives, and as the site wherein other narratives take place.[1] To the extent that local populations are conflated with place, they take on each other's characteristics; that is, as populations are totalized, they may become both a single entity or character and also a passive site of the actions of characters whose relations to place may be rather complicated. In turn, as places are personified, they take on the character of actors (in the Burkean sense) with motives and stories of their own. This is most obviously dramatized in novels and plays like Jerrold's *History of St. James and St. Giles,* in which individuals are given the names and characteristics of places, but it is also more subtly evidenced—and with more effective force on policy making—in the narratives of moral environmentalism with that characteristic villain, "the deleterious place."

It is this logic which was in part evident in the public reception of the New Oxford Street cut, which razed the Rookery, a notorious Irish slum dwelling that became the emblem of St. Giles. The assumption was that in destroying the space, the problem would be solved. Yet, as much subsequent testimony showed, there was little thought about the problem of the people who lived in the Rookery who therefore were simply concentrated into an even smaller number of available lodging houses in the surrounding area. Typically, this failure was often blamed by journalists and policy makers alike on the "character" of St. Giles and the "peculiar habits" of the people who lived there—despite the fact that such slums existed all over the city and its environs. The parishes of St. Giles in the Fields and St. James's, Westminster, physically in close proximity to each other yet traditionally opposite economically and socially, together were often used to symbolize London's ability to contain extremes within the close confines of the urban landscape. The operation of such a perception can perhaps best be seen when an event occurs which challenges it. The cholera epidemic of 1854, which was in part constructed as an inversion of the relationship between the two parishes, was such an event.

The story of the paired places St. James's and St. Giles* is always a kinship narrative. The parishes are figured as twins, and when they are so invoked, their meaning is different from the symbolism evoked by each singly. St. Giles alone meant poverty, squalor, and the Irish slums, just as Whitechapel meant poverty, squalor, and Jewish slums, whereas St. James's alone still meant the pomp and splendor of court. However, St. James's and Whitechapel would never have been yoked together, although they stood in a similar economic relation as St. James's and St. Giles. Geographic proximity is part of the relation, as is history, and perhaps also the invocation of the sister isles of England and Ireland (just as West and East London often invoked England and its Eastern possessions). The alliteration of the names is also an important part of the tendency to fit the two parishes into a structure of kinship stories—a tradition of twin conflict myths in which the goodness of one depends upon the counterbalancing evil of the other. In fact, within this structure, for the existence of the good twin, there must be the evil one—urban industrialism's Mr. Hyde. St. Giles had long been associated with epidemic disease, and large numbers of deaths there in 1832 and the late 1840s only confirmed this association, as did St. James's relative exemption from illness reinforce the connection between wealth and health.

The city, especially the capital city and metropole, exists simultaneously as a real space, with real topographies filled with people having lived experiences of that space—the *parole* of urban life—and as a mythic place, a perceived space for consumption not only of urban dwellers but of the national/imperial subject, a myth whose specifically metropolitan logic must be mapped onto a sometimes recalcitrant natural, built, and lived environment.[2] The urban ethnography as a genre from the 1840s through the 1860s participated in and helped shape and perpetuate mythic narratives about race, evolution, moral environmentalism, and so forth. Within that framework, it is not surprising that St. James's would be the place of whiteness, lightness, Englishness, and cleanliness (while simultaneously representing the entire Empire—hence the crystal palace and the Exhibition), while St. Giles would be the place of racial degeneration, darkness (dark alleys and stifling rooms), Irishness, and filth. St. James's, in short, was widely perceived to be the ideal space conceived by sanitarians and urban planners, whereas St. Giles represented its opposite.

An imagined national community requires at least a hazy notion of a mapped place, with margins (India, as we shall see in chapters 6 and 7, offered

*In naming the parishes, I have followed common mid-Victorian usage. In most documents, St. James's parish was generally referred to as St. James's, whereas most referred to St. Giles without the possessive. I have retained this usage, except in instances wherein, in quoted material, the writer deviated from the norm.

an important site for those defining differences) and a center or metropole. (The margins may change easily without much damage to the idea of the nation; the center, rarely. The most significant attempt at such a recuperation may be Augustine's *City of God*, and even he does not suggest a new material site, only a symbolic one.) The metropole must not only represent the richness and diversity of its nation, but contain it. The literature and journalism of nineteenth-century Britain was primarily metropolitan in both concern and content. Yet it also represented that metropole to thousands who had never seen it, or had never seen all of it, or who lived in it and yet experienced it as a lived space in a manner which did not adequately render London as the idea of the metropole.

For these readers, London could be rendered in two manners: first in the manner of a travelogue, with specific descriptions, routes, and addresses—a utilitarian rendition of specific places, and second, as a place definable by a few symbolic spaces and pairings—Westminster Abbey, London Bridge, and the like, or East End-West End, St. James's and St. Giles—symbolic shorthand having less to do with real places than with the imaginal containment of differences too rich to be grasped in their multiplicity. Even for city dwellers who knew these places well, there are levels of discourse in which it is appropriate to identify, say, Chelsea, as "London," the "West End," or "Chelsea" or even perhaps "Cheyne Walk," depending on one's audience, purpose, and so forth. But even Londoners who knew their city well seem to have read St. Giles as the Rookery and St. James's as the Palace and the Mall, not only in contexts in which those parishes were clearly being invoked, not as places, but as symbols, but also too often in attempting to deal with individual dwellers of individual places within the two parishes. Whereas in the seventeenth century a slum might simply have meant a dangerous or undesirable place, or even the downside of urban life, in the nineteenth century, St. Giles, always described as situated in the heart of London, represented the moral failure of the British nation in a way that a slum in Manchester, no matter how foul, never did. In fact, as Alan Bewell argues, such spaces represented the incursion of a "tropical" colonial geography, with its imaginary entailments of darkness, moisture, crowding, fever, and stifling heat. As we have seen in the last chapter, the filth of the slum was associated with a barbaric past, out of which the nation must progress; St. Giles became a byword for this embarrassing barbarism to be eliminated, just as St. James's represented the pinnacle of metropolitan wealth and sophistication.[3]

If the city, especially the metropolis, operates as a particular kind of myth, it must mediate between the open systems of history and lived topography and the closed system of symbolic activity—the parish as a static node of meaning. The tendency to see, for example, the entire parish of St. Giles and its multifarious population of individuals as metonymically represented by the Rookery, even after its destruction, provides an excellent example of the way in which moral environmentalism works with the perception of urban topography as continuous and meaningful space (rather than as a large heterogenous space broken up into neighborhoods, individual houses, and so on) to deemphasize the individual and the smaller community in favor of an aggregate which the parish comes first to represent, and then to supplant. Working from an understanding of human experience as storied, if we see places as narrative elements caught up in multiple coexisting narratives, we can begin to see the elements which make up the story of London and of St. James's and St. Giles—a story powerful enough to resist the incursion of a counternarrative of fact even in the face of so disturbing an event as a cholera epidemic. This story would have to be reconciled with other narratives, including those extending from the newer knowledges associated with medical geography and statistics.

Initially, one might see this as a conflict between a temporal form (narrative) and a spatial one (medical geography), but of course, medical geography, as we have seen, is itself embedded in various narratives of evolution, progress, and so on. I have been using the term "myth" here to refer to a type of narrative in which time tends to be static or cyclic and narrative elements tend to be perceived as representing types rather than individuals, and I shall continue to use the term "myth" throughout as shorthand for this mode of narration. However, another way to consider this dichotomy is as the opposition which obtains between melodrama and realism—melodrama proceeding according to class and moral category and accounting for difference by reducing it again to type (the beautiful and pure poor girl turns out to be nobly born after all), in which characters are relatively static, and realism, which oscillates between type and individual to engage a vision of progress (or decline) in social and self-development. My point here is not to suggest that there are pure mythic/melodramatic or realist genres—these are better described as modes of narration embedded within texts that usually contain multiple modes. But as Nancy Armstrong has made clear, there is at least a rough parallel between the emergence of what she calls the modern individual in domestic fiction, or what would become high Victorian realism, which first coexisted with earlier narrative forms which were less focused on individual self-development and the potential for change, and eventually moved them increasingly into the domain of popular culture.

This shift, then, is in part as a mediation between an older class-based categorization of individuals (where class is essential, rather than contingent) and one based on the body and its practices, which the practice of public health of course sees as malleable (otherwise, what would be the point of melioration?). In the first vision, the poor are always with us, and always (already) dirty and diseased; the salient classificatory characteristic is class. In the second, individuals can change, all are potential citizens, potentially clean and proper bodies, and all are equally potential victims of disease, which becomes not a feature of subjectivity, but of circumstance, landscape. It is, then, not a matter of moving from abstract typology to specificity, but of moving from a relatively fixed typology based on one or two characteristics (class, for example, or the humoral body) to a much broader typology based on the modern, malleable body, out of which, in turn, it is possible to fragment the now much larger abstract class based on other contingencies which are not seen as essential (what well one drinks at, for example).[4]

Sanitary science began this shift, but was still broadly based on the older mode of narration—geographic characteristics which acted on the body were themselves class based and produced by the bodies they acted upon. Dirt and drunkenness were produced by the poor because they desired them. But the sanitarian paradigm opened the possibility of thinking of a universal standard of health in which the dirt and drunkenness of the poor was not natural, but a perversion of nature. This in turn opened the way to a medical realist model of the equivalence of bodies and the understanding that, just as the poor were no more naturally dirty and diseased than the rich, the rich were not naturally but situationally immune from dirt and disease, and that situations were subject to change, as they had in St. James's. The mythic pairing of healthy, wealthy (English) St. James's and poor, sick (foreign) St. Giles gives way to a model which can account for the heterogeneity of outcomes during the epidemic, in which all bodies are basically assumed to be equal and the difference emerges from circumstance rather than class characteristics. And medical knowledges—geography, vital statistics, and so forth—provide these alternative narratives. In turn, these narratives provide ways of meliorating the cholera that are unavailable within the other narrative structure. They also, as we have seen, disrupted the primacy of the parish as the unit of population identity. So the parish as individual actor (elegant St. James's, vile St. Giles) would eventually become instead potentially heterogenous communities in which one's membership in a particular community organized around medical-geographic factors which could cross parish boundaries, but might extend only one or two streets, or might extend the entire length of a particular waterway.

Returning to the use of parish-as-actor, parish identity had much to do with perceived history. If St. James's history had been written as the story of kings and queens—of individuals who, in themselves, represented communities and nations—St. Giles' history is written as the history of the aggregate—of the Irish, of prostitutes, of thieves: a history of plurals. Even the individuals who are hauled up for our inspection by such meticulous chroniclers as Mayhew are representative of the aggregate: a "water cress girl" who is quickly appropriated and reused by Mayhew's imitators. Poovey suggests that it is in the 1830s that techniques of social control insistently position lower-class individuals as a massed aggregate to be treated as a passive whole in policymaking. Certainly, we see this aggregate conflated with and represented by place.

Inevitably, in the emerging commodity culture of the mid-nineteenth century (which recent historians have argued was consolidated by, or perhaps even began with the Great Exhibition of 1851) places became intensely commodified, often as tourist attractions. Whereas real estate value had always been defined by space—fortuitous geographical location, views, convenience to the city, and so on—as well as by fashion, place-names now became even more important as tourism, travel narratives, and local ethnographies were, more than ever, significant ways in which the London experience was apprehended.[5] In reading spaces, public places are more likely to define a place than private ones, those associated with wealth and power are more important than those identified with modest means, and ones that are centrally located and highly visible are more likely to become keys for the urban reader than inaccessible or marginal ones; history also affects the branding of places.[6]

The actual histories of the two parishes, as well as their locations, had much to do with their identities as intimate opposites. The history of St. Giles in the Fields as a plague spot had been of long standing, and preceded its incorporation into the physical boundaries of the city. The church was founded in 1101, substantially to the west of urban London, as the chapel of a hospital for lepers, by Matilda, queen to Henry I. Although the lepers who lived there were the daughters of wealthy families, leprosy itself was associated with Jews and with lustful and intemperate habits. Sir Rowland Dobie's meticulous history of St. Giles, written in 1834, refers to leprosy in the twelfth century in rather familiar terms: "Among the Jews, it [leprosy] existed to a formidable degree. . . . [T]he exact nature of the malady has been much questioned; there is, however, little doubt but its inveteracy was engendered by uncleanliness—dirty linen—and want of baths during their wanderings in the desarts [sic]" (5).

In the mid-sixteenth century the colony became a parish church, ministering to the village of St. Giles. By the mid-seventeenth century, it seems to have become a part of the western boundary of London, and it is in 1664 that St. Giles became the vector for the plague, the first cases having occurred there in November. Dobie quotes the legendary physician Sydenham as making the connection between poverty and plague: "'This plague . . . discovered its first malignity among the poorer sort of people in St. Giles'" (130). Additionally, St. Giles Church had the distinction of being the last stop in the pilgrimage of condemned criminals before their execution at Tyburn. Dobie also notes that, according to parish records, the Irish were associated with St. Giles as far back as Elizabeth I (192), who decreed that no more buildings should be raised, thus inadvertently insuring that overcrowding would be the result, although this observation may say more about Dobie's interest in finding historical materials to confirm his own perceptions than the reality of life in St. Giles in Elizabethan times. However, Hogarth does set his gin palaces in St. Giles, and many eighteenth-century references confirm that St. Giles was then considered a resort of low characters. Although, according to Gordon Taylor, it had been considered "one of the fashionable places to live" in the seventeenth century (13), "[f]rom about 1750 the parish of St. Giles slowly became a byword for poverty and squalor" (14).

By the nineteenth century, the perception of St. Giles as Irish slum and moral and physical plague spot was very well established. Today a part of the borough of Holborn, the boundaries of the large and irregularly *L*-shaped mid-nineteenth-century parish extended from Francis Street to Tottenham Court Road, followed that road down to Crown Street, curved down West Street and onto Castle Street to include the notorious Seven Dials area, followed Castle to Drury Lane, meandered around to take in Lincoln's Inn Fields and half of Lincoln's Inn Gardens, ambled back up High Holborn to Broad Street and extended upward to include the area somewhat north of and including Bedford Square. It curved around St. George's, Bloomsbury and also abutted St. Anne's Soho, St. Martin's, St. Andrew's, St. Clement's, and St. Pancras. The parish included a variable population, but was best known for the Rookery (also known as the "Holyland" because of its Irish Catholic population) located at the bend of the L, not far from Seven Dials. As one nineteenth-century commentator put it:

> The hospital passed away, but upon its site arose the church and village of St. Giles; and then the great city, stretching out its polypus' arms, seized upon the village, and, drawing it to her bosom, crushed out its healthy life in the powerful embrace.
>
> The hospital has disappeared, but it has left its seal upon the spot, and lepers by the thousand crowd where the lazar-house has been—lepers, but no longer standing afar off, without the gates of cities, scattering dust upon their heads. . . . But, herding together, they throw aside the garment that hides their shame, and rejoice in the leprosy of ignorance and sin which isolates them from their kind—a leprosy never absent from places such as these, the head-quarters of indigence and filth—a leprosy which incrusts from head to heel the inhabitants of this quondam village of St. Giles. (in a printed piece pasted in on page 24 of Dobie, on which page is recorded Henry the VIII's dissolution of the hospital)

St. Giles's sufferings during the first two cholera epidemics far exceeded surrounding areas, which of course, was exactly what was expected of it.

St. James's parish began its history as St. Giles's twin indeed. It was founded, well outside of London, shortly after St. Giles was, and was also a leper colony. According to Burford, the leper hospital (also for women) was founded in or just after 1117, and remained so until 1450, when it was changed to a convent (1–3). It was in 1532 that its fortunes changed, when Henry VIII purchased the convent and erected a summer dwelling and hunting lodge, and also enclosed the grounds which were to become St. James Park. The existence of an important royal dwelling in St. James's would alter the ways in which it could be perceived. As the city grew to meet St. James Palace and its environs, it became more and more a part of court life leading to the erection of stately homes, the famous theaters, the coffee houses and clubs with which we have come to associate the image of St. James's in the late seventeenth and eighteenth century. St. James's was, of course, also notorious as the site of whorehouses and low entertainments in this period, but they were low entertainments at least partly for highly placed people. By Victoria's reign, St. James Palace was used for all ceremonial and state occasions, including the royal wedding, despite her residence in Buckingham Palace (Glasheen), and the parish of St. James's, whatever its variegated history, was a symbolic center and locus amoenus of London and Britain.

As may well be imagined, the success of St. James's insured that its neighbor would not enjoy similar distinction; indeed the outer reaches of St. James's which bordered St. Giles was the Drury Lane theater and entertainment district, which provided for the existence of parasitic slums. Within St. James's, by the mid-nineteenth century, the poor areas were, according to sanitary and census reports, mostly populated by workers devoted to the rag trade, whereas St. Giles was the resort of costermongers and flower sellers as well as pickpockets and prostitutes, as Mayhew so memorably chronicled.

St. James's, although actually part of the City of Westminster, rather than technically the City of London, clearly represented (Greater) London as the metropolitan seat of power to Victorian British subjects. In turn, it represented Great Britain to foreigners as well. With the approach of the Great Exhibition, Londoners had an even keener than usual sense of civic, national, and metropolitan pride. Finally becoming, in their own regard, comparable to the great city across the channel, Londoners were inspired by the coming exhibition, as a display of national might, to read their city critically through foreign eyes. While St. James's was the pride of the English, notwithstanding those questionable areas that did not easily come into view from the main thoroughfares, St. Giles became the symbol of national embarrassment. Having borne a disproportionate burden of attention as an image of the dark side of metropolitan life in the national press, St. Giles became a negative tourist attraction for foreigners wishing to see the slums of London without the inconvenience of East End travel. In 1850, Charles Purton Cooper writes to Sir George Greg, M.P.,

Sir, that part of the parish of St. Giles in the Fields to which the ensuing papers relate is beginning to attract the attention of foreigners anxious to acquire information respecting our social position in all its parts—the bad as well as the good. [In September and October, it was visited by several foreigners, among them three French and two Americans from New York.]. . . . It is not necessary that you should have the mortification of reading the remarks, which I have had the mortification of hearing. My object may be attained without the infliction of that pain [but St. Giles is unaltered and, without intervention, will remain so at the opening of the Exhibition next year]. . . . The curiosity of strangers with respect to the spot in question—little at the present moment—may then grow great; the human mind is apt to delight in contrasts—and how humiliating will be the consequence, not only to the inhabitants of our metropolis, but to Englishmen generally, is abundantly obvious. (5–6)

Indeed, St. Giles had been an object of foreign interest for some time. The *Revue des Deux Mondes,* not without a certain malice, published an entire series on the worst parishes in London, including Whitechapel and Liverpool, but the long article by Léon Faucher, reprinted as extracts and sold in tract form, on St. Giles was perhaps the most damning:

À Londres, le quartier par excéllence des gens sans aveu est la paroisse de Saint-Giles, lieu célèbre dans les fastes criminels, qu'habitent concurrement avec les vagabonds irlandais les prostituées de bas étage et les voleurs de profession. Saint-Giles figure en pâté de rues étroites, d'allées sombres et de cours fétides, situé dans l'angle que foment, derrière la cathédrale de Saint-Paul et au coeur de la Cité, les deux grandes voies de Londres. (Faucher 4)

Faucher concludes, "Si l'Angleterre a jamais humilie quelque grande nation, ce peuple n'a qu'à regarder Londres, et il se trouvera trop vengé" (Faucher 31).

St. Giles's central location also contributed to its significance as a blot on the city's luster, as suggested above. The fact that it was close to such attractions as the British Museum meant that it was far more likely to be seen, even by visitors not seeking such thrills, than the slums farther east. The popular shilling guidebook *A Week in London* mentions only one slum, St. Giles, in the context of directions for a walk from the British Museum: "Forming a continuation of Holborn . . . is Broad Street, St. Giles . . . occupied by the very lowest class of society and through which it is hardly safe to pass alone even in the day-time" (24). Dickens, of course, had long since done much to popularize the image of St. Giles in the *Sketches by Boz* as "filthy and miserable. . . . [It] can hardly be imagined by those . . . who have not witnessed it. Wretched houses with broken windows . . . starvation in the attics, Irishmen in the passage, a "musician" in the front kitchen, and a charwoman with five hungry children in the back one—filth everywhere" (212–13).[7] Throughout the period, St. Giles is constantly referred to as the paradigmatic slum.

Thomas Beames's 1850 volume *The Rookeries of London, Past, Present and Prospective* begins with two chapters on general definitions of rookeries and their development, and then devotes his first case study chapter to St. Giles: "In common parlance, St. Giles's and Billingsgate are types—the one, of the lowest conditions under which human life is possible,—the other, of the lowest point to which the English language can descend" (19). After some animadversions on the Rookery (also, evidently, a type) and its demolition some years before, Beames provides a detailed description of the remaining slums (that is, the area surrounding the New Oxford Cut) in George Street and Church Lane, into which the residents of the former Rookery have been driven: "[T]urn aside from streets whose shops teem with every luxury—where Art has brought together its most beautiful varieties,—and you have scarce gone a hundred yards when you are in 𝕿𝖍𝖊 𝕽𝖔𝖔𝖐𝖊𝖗𝖞. The change is marvellous: squalid children, haggard men, with long uncombed hair, in rags, most of them smoking, many speaking Irish; women without shoes or stockings—a babe perhaps at the breast, with a single garment, confined to the waist by a bit of string, wolfish looking dogs" (30).

It is important to notice to what extent slum conditions are referred to as the Irishness of the population; from noting the presence of Irish residents, the slum itself comes to represent the presence of Irish population until it practically becomes a causal relationship reflecting the troubled relations of Ireland to the Kingdom: the slum becomes, finally a synecdoche for Irishness and by extension for Ireland itself. Beames's solution for this is that

> Rookeries, at least such as Church Lane, should be proscribed; it would be difficult, with our free institutions, to stop these descents of Irish upon our Great Towns; but the names of those who land here should be entered in a book, their progress observed, and, if they did not get work within a certain time, they should be sent back to their own Unions. [. . .] The misery, filth, and crowded condition of an Irish cabin, is realised in St. Giles's. (38)

Kearns and Philo suggest, "It might be argued that the black inner city becomes the focus of what, following Said's example, can be termed an 'imaginative geography.' . . . [W]hat is projected on to both the people and their place is indeed a sense of 'distance and difference': a sense perhaps of being alien, wild, promiscuous, irreligious, unrestrained and diseased . . . and where the physical decay of the built environment is taken as a reflection of—and maybe as actually being caused by—the cultural shortcomings of the black inhabitants" (31). Certainly this was the case for many London residents in the nineteenth century, with the substitution of the Irish slums of St. Giles and Southwark (and perhaps the Jewish one of Whitechapel) for today's urban underclass. In fact, after Mayhew, there was a surge of local journalism which treated London slums as "safari territory," producing ethnographies which charted the behaviors of the "natives" often in specifically colonial terms: "The women here are perhaps more vicious than the men. The people crowded about were more dangerous and savage than a tribe of Caffres" (newsprint, pasted in Dobie, dated Jan. 10, 1863).

Peter J. Keating, among others, has argued that the literature of sanitary reform in the midcentury, which was widely distributed and eagerly read, incorporated both elements of colonial exploration literature turned inward, with its metaphor of "deepest, darkest London."[8] Certainly this genre of publication contributed to the consumption of London slums as a kind of safari commodity. Foreign tourists of London slums may also have been moved by a desire to undercut the supremacy of London in its boasted status as center of the world, at least in their own consumption of it. This impulse toward imaginative geography, howsoever motivated, was as powerful a means of selling places—at least for touristic consumption, as the more deliberate ones (although it may certainly have been less effective as capitalist enterprise). In any case, to Londoners, the British, and perhaps the world, St. Giles represented the failure of the nation, just as St. James's represented its brilliance.

With these perceptions of the two parishes firmly in place, the challenge posed by the events of 1854 was shocking. The cholera, a disease which struck quickly in epidemic form and killed many in the course of a few months before subsiding, foregrounded civic tensions, as dramatic public events do.[9] Again, as with all public events, the cholera epidemics were understood within narratives which were combined and reconciled with existing narratives about class, race, urban life, nation, and place. By the mid-1850s, two previous epidemics had struck London (in 1832 and in 1849) and had established geographical patterns which seemed to reinforce contemporary notions of moral environmentalism. The cause of cholera being unknown, susceptibility to the disease was ascribed to moral degeneracy from the first epidemic on. In 1832, it was thought to be the special scourge of drunkards and blasphemers. The poor generally were suspect, and the poor Irish, regarded as naturally dirty, came under particular scrutiny in the late 1840s and 1850s, especially with regard to their funeral practices and the celebration of wakes.

Despite the objections of many doctors, who ascribed the impact of the disease largely to environmental factors rather than personal habits, this perception of epidemic disease causation continued to dominate among the general public until late in the century. As the disease took hold, often killing children and occasionally killing in the respectable middle class, the onus of immorality was ascribed less to individuals than to a local population, especially one which could be racially defined such as the Irish. In this way the deaths of blameless individuals could be reconciled with the sense of moral responsibility accruing to a degenerate, diseased population in a diseased location, individuals being elided in favor of an aggregate, and then the aggregate being elided again in favor of a place which came to stand for the habits of the population.

A typical example of this logic can be found in one of John Sutherland's 1852 reports:

> It is the result of observation, that if dwellings be ever so bad, there will still be people found of a character similar to the dwellings to inhabit them. I have observed this so often that I consider it an established law in civic economy; and it is a most important one, for it points out the remedies required. . . . Unhealthy localities attract certain classes of people, and overcrowding renders cleanliness and ventilation very difficult, even if the people were disposed to put them into operation. Unhealthy houses act upon the people, and the people re-act upon the houses, and thus cause and effect are interchanged, and the result is disease mortality, demoralization and crime. (5–6)

Cholera was a filth disease, filthy people were immoral, the Irish were filthy, and cholera killed most savagely in Irish slums. St. Giles had long been a byword as an Irish slum and even longer as a seat of disease, and St. Giles had suffered heavy mortality rates in the first two epidemics. The 1854 visitation changed this pattern. For the first time, St. James's, practically untouched by the first two epidemics, saw far heavier mortality than ever before, and much more than its dark twin.

Anglican clergy and various liberal factions, each for its own reasons, seized the opportunity to comment on the essential fraternity of humanity in their vulnerability to disease. Although the clergy had contributed historically to the perception of cholera as a visitation of God's wrath, the Anglican Church having in 1832 declared the cholera a punishment for "national sins," by the midcentury both they and liberal sanitarians wished to impress upon the general population their moral responsibility to the classes most likely to die of cholera, in order that some prophylactic and charitable intervention might take place. To this end, a peculiar combination of rhetoric was used to excite both pity for the miserable conditions under which the poor lived, and fear that the filthy dwellings would have such a demoralizing effect that the lower classes might rise against the upper, both individually, as burglars and pickpockets, and socially, in revolutionary movements. Both groups stressed the vulnerability of the upper classes to the lower (a rhetoric which makes the charity of the upper classes look more like protection money), and the deaths of St. James's residents, imagined as wealthy or at least respectable, enabled these concerns to be expressed more forcefully in terms of epidemiological vulnerability as well. Put another way, both groups were mobilizing an existing mythic narrative, and the challenge put to it by recent events, for suasive purposes. A typical response comes to hand in Rev. Henry Venn Elliott's 1854 sermon:

> [F]amiliarity with the scourge in a milder form took off the terror, till the disease, whether endemic or epidemic, came to be regarded as one which might, to a considerable extent, be provided against by public and private precautions. Cleanliness . . . and an early application of medicine and medical skill . . . were supposed to be specifics against the contagion. And to a certain extent there is some truth in these views; and it is thus that God enforces on us, by his great and invariable laws of health, the necessity of attention to these sanitary measures. . . . Then the selfishness of our nature, leaving the poor in their disease or in their danger to pay the penalty of their localities, was heard to congratulate itself on the comparative safety of its better situations. . . . And then it was . . . that the cholera at one leap passed from the squalid abodes of poverty into the houses which were rejoicing in their comforts, and the streets which were high and clean. No districts, I hear, have suffered more from the cholera than certain parts of the parish of St. James's, and in certain vicinities of Oxford-street and Soho-square. . . . These events put an end to the fancied and selfish security of the healthier parts of London. (9–11)

The horrifying inexplicability of the disease's volte-face in its customary habits is suggested in the formal report of the Cholera Inquiry Committee, which stresses again and again that there was neither topographical nor economic consistency in the outbreak:

> It is this startling suddenness of the outbreak that has given it a scientific interest, scarcely less momentous than its social importance; and as few of us probably will ever witness its like again, it is most desirable that no pains should be spared in its thorough investigation. . . . Some narrow streets and courts suffered severely; others nearly or quite escaped, as Tyler's, Great Crown and Walker's Courts; whilst wide streets, as Broad Street itself, were heavily visited. . . . A want of cleanliness in streets or houses was be no means a constant accompaniment of the disease. Some houses in the midst of others affected escaped, without any favorable sanitary condition. . . . On the whole it would appear that the disease did not limit its attack to any one class, nor yet to the very poor. (*Report . . . St. James's* 24–31)

Indeed, it would seem that many residents holding onto the class-bound, melodramatic vision of epidemiology were unwilling to believe that they had been struck by the cholera at all—it must be some other disease which had so decimated the inhabitants of St. James's, though throughout England, and indeed, most of Europe, cholera raged: "[I]t has often been alleged that in some way or other the remains of decomposing animal matter, or indeed the plague matter itself, lying in the soil of this district, are chargeable with the great mortality from Cholera near it. Popular opinion has even gone so far as to maintain that the disease of last autumn was not Cholera, but a direful kind of black fever" (*Report . . . St. James's* 46). However, the report argues against this interpretation. After extensive discussion of the Lord Craven pest fields, cemetery pits from the time of the plague, supposed to lie under part of the parish, part of which is under Broad Street, the report concludes that they can have had little effect. Why, after all, was St. James's spared in the previous two epidemics, when the plague matter was younger and therefore more potentially injurious? John Snow also notes the prevalence of local belief in this explanation:

> Many persons were inclined to attribute the severity of the malady in this locality to the very circumstance to which some people attribute the comparative immunity of the city of London from the same disease, viz., to the drains in the neighborhood having been disturbed and put in about half a year previously. . . . Many of the non-medical public were disposed to attribute the outbreak of cholera to the supposed existence of a pit in which persons dying of the plague had been buried about two centuries ago; and, if the alleged plague-pit had been nearer to Broad Street, they would no doubt still cling to the idea. The situation of the pit, however, is said to be Little Marlborough Street, just out of the area in which the chief mortality occurred. With regard to effluvia from the sewers passing into the streets and houses, that is a fault common to most parts of London and other towns. (*On the Mode* 54–55)

Another rumor, which the General Board of Health reports had "gone the round of the papers, to the effect that the vast majority of the deaths occurred in the upper rooms" and therefore weren't householders but lodgers or servants (Fraser, Hughes, and Ludlow 155), reflects again the belief that cholera was a disease of the poor. The board, however, concludes that this was not the case.

It is clear that residents were unwilling to believe explanations that challenged the existing notions of causality, which may have provided a comforting sense of containment for what otherwise must have seemed horrifically inexplicable. Yet, it was probably easier to believe that they had been poisoned by the bodily products of their poorer neighbors than it was to believe that St. James's residents might in fact be those poorer neighbors. As David Harvey has noted, "The geography of human activity in large metropolitan areas appears to generate curious transformations and inversions to create a complex geography of subjective class-consciousness" which has little to do with actual economic or working status (*Urbanization of Capital* 83). Here, people living in poverty comparable to much worse areas gain respectability in large part from their location. However unwilling Londoners were to accept that St. James's had truly been stricken by the cholera, its presence in St. James's allowed more awareness of the range of individual cases involved and the vulnerability of respectable working people to the disease. In fact, as an examination of London Cholera Hospital casebooks from 1832 shows, the disease had always stricken many steady working people of temperate habits, a fact that had eluded the public understanding of the disease.

The vulnerability of respectable working-class people in St. James's so thoroughly contradicted what was believed about the disease that the Cholera Inquiry Committee threw up its hands and tentatively suggested that John Snow's explanation was about as good a one as they were likely to find (St. James's 71). The outbreak in St. James's probably did far more to advance Snow's credibility than his meticulous research did. Others also evinced unwillingness to believe that such a disease could really strike equally across class lines. Even during the epidemic, the *Times* argued that

> persons of all ranks and of every degree of affluence were attacked and died. But it will immediately be seen that the poor in London suffered greater losses from cholera than the rich. . . . Over every district of London, both classes are distributed, . . . and among the poor, though not in any way belonging to the industrious classes, are a mixed, idle, intemperate, dirty, wretched, and often criminal class, who are dwelling in courts and lanes not far from the mansions of the wealthy. ("Cholera" 7)

Here again, the peculiarity of high death rates in St. James's, as opposed to low ones in Bethnal Green, is also explained by Snow's theory on the impurity of water sources, which is somehow to be incorporated into existing moral environmentalism, perhaps as the anomaly that proves the rule, but at the expense of the coherence of place identity.

We see here an attempt to retain the mythic view of epidemiology, but without the mythic view of place that underpins it. In short, a number of strategies were attempted to mediate between the mythic view of epidemiology promoted by sanitary science, which was supported by equally melodramatic narratives of place and the realist view associated with medical visions of the social body. Some tried to hold on to one without losing the other, as seen above. However, since epidemiology had been conceptualized as a spatial knowledge, it was quite difficult to continue to tell a melodramatic, class-bound story of the disease without recourse to that view of place. And once place lost its coherence and identity, becoming abstracted and recategorized by realist narratives of medical geography, it was increasingly difficult to hang onto older narratives of epidemiology. Once place was restructured, bodies also, eventually, had to be narrated differently—as structurally equivalent, rather than essentially classed.

Obviously, it took a while for this contradiction to work through, and thus, the incoherencies of arguments in which the laws of health decree that there is some logic to imagining oneself immune if one lives in a healthy, clean neighborhood, but in which those laws of general providence may be broken by the special providence of God seeking to punish those who then draw the obvious conclusion that the poor may be left to their own devices. Those who did not have recourse to the religious argument—which changes the narrative rules by simply overriding the logic of the sanitary explanation while still declaring it generally valid—were forced either to throw up their hands in defeat or to cling to the medical theory of Snow or the sanitary theory at the expense of St. James's reputation. These last were absolutely right about the distribution of poverty in the city, and the sanitary explanation was therefore absolutely functional in the case of this epidemic. But, fortunately, the melodrama of place was sufficiently powerful to override the weaker melodrama of sanitary science (weaker because it already provided logically for its opposite), thus enabling the medical-geographic explanation of cholera's epidemiology play. Ironically, of course, this new vision of space ultimately would undermine the traditional melodrama of place which defined St. James's and St. Giles.

As we have seen, Snow had argued his theory of cholera as early as 1849. Using statistics from all over the city, he paid particular attention to an outbreak very similar to the St. James's one, in Wandsworth, where a similarly shocking death rate had concentrated in a small area. Hector Gavin notes in his sanitary report of 1848 that Wandsworth was one of the two healthiest districts in London, according to Metropolitan Returns, but it was to suffer extremely heavily shortly after this and Snow made it the occasion of his first detailed personal investigation into the sewage-contaminated water theory. Although it drew the attention of Farr and other epidemiologists, it received relatively little widespread attention, and from the point of view of the general public, the anomalous Wandsworth epidemic may as well have never taken place. St. James's, however, the glamorous parish in the heart of the city, was literally another story. As we saw in the last chapter, the Board of Health, the General Registrar's Office, the Royal College of Physicians, the parish vestry, and, of course, Snow himself, all published book-length studies of the outbreak, and many more sermons and pamphlets on the topic were circulated. The St. James's outbreak bids fair to be the most investigated epidemic incident in London's history; it certainly is the single most investigated incident in London of any of the four cholera epidemics.

The naming of the epidemic is also significant. Despite the fact that this is as often called the Golden Square outbreak as the Broad Street outbreak (when it is not simply called the St. James's outbreak), there were very few deaths anywhere near the more or less respectable Golden Square address itself, and the Golden Square registration district suffered proportionately with the adjacent Berwick Street registration district. Snow does map two deaths right across the street from Golden Square, but in the greater detail of the board's map—three times the size of the Snow map—we see one death there, oriented toward upper John Street (that is, around the corner from, rather than facing Golden Square), and that is within a building marked "Homeopathic Hospital." Berwick Street, on the other hand, was known as a seedy area; the curate of St. Luke's, Berwick Street, is the only writer I have found who references the epidemic as a "Berwick Street" event. Golden Square became a reference point that highlighted again the horror of such an event taking place in St. James's, near public areas associated with wealth and the consumption of luxury goods. As far away as Brighton, Rev. Henry Venn Elliott marveled to his congregation, many of whom had fled unhealthy London to this fashionable watering hole, "It is stated that in Broad-street *[sic]*, which has fifty houses, and which is reached from Oxford street by only one short street, there were deaths in every house but one on the south side" (10). Clearly, St. James's as a reference point mobilized more public identification and interest than poor Wandsworth. And St. Giles's comparative immunity could not but be particularly stunning in the light of St. James's suffering.

In fact, despite the difference in the fortunes of the twins, the composition of the two parishes in the mid-nineteenth century were not so widely at variance as the myth would suggest. The public perception of the 1854 epidemic highlights the way in which the myth of cholera as a disease or moral and physical degeneracy was pitted against the mythic reading of St. James's. An analysis of the facts indicates that the myth of cholera as a slum disease was entirely consistent with the facts of the mortality in St. James's. However, it was inconsistent with St. James's as perceived space. It is this perception which succeeds over both fact and cholera myth, and which enabled Snow to gain a more sympathetic hearing for his theory than he might otherwise have received.

Upon examination, it is clear that the two parishes, in many neighborhoods not significantly economically at variance, were misread to be consistent with the myth. In an interesting gesture, George Buchanan, the medical officer for St. Giles, concedes that, per capita, St. Giles is really quite comparable to neighboring parishes in terms of wealth, but for his own specifically sanitary purposes, he performs a most interesting racial calculus to make his observations conform to the widely held image of St. Giles:

> The amount assessed on each district to the county-rate, divided by the population, gives also a useful idea of the relative richness or poverty of a district. Thus examined, St. Giles is poorer than some, but richer than other of its neighbors. . . . [But it is more important for a health officer] to be aware of the actual amount of the very lowest and poorest that it contains, for these are the persons among whom disease is chiefly engendered and perpetuated.

Without disparagement to our sister island, which seems to produce alike the noblest and the lowest in the social scale, it must be confessed that the relative numbers of Irish [listed at twenty percent on page 31, highest in the surrounding area] in our London districts, will furnish no bad gauge of the extremity of poverty. . . . As far, therefore, as it is fair to regard the numbers of Irish as a test of poverty, St. Giles is shown to contain more of the extremely poor than any of the surrounding districts. (32)

Although St. Giles, because it had a few very notorious slums contained within the parish (which were indeed very overcrowded and in which people indeed lived under appalling conditions), had become a byword for poverty, crime and filth, St. James's, like most parishes, had its share of slums as well. Although those living in St. James's poor areas were more likely to be steadily employed, often the conditions under which they lived were nearly if not actually as bad as those of more casual laborers in far more notorious slums such as Seven Dials. In an 1847 tract the author complains of inadequate sewage throughout St. James's, remarking that the greater part of Piccadilly was, before 1841, "without a sewer at all," relying entirely on cesspools ("An Address" 5). Further, the author points out, there were within a small area of the parish in 1847 fourteen overcrowded cowsheds, two slaughterhouses, three boiling houses and seven bones stores, all of which tended to contribute to a noxious sanitary environment, a description which matches information from other sources. The author quotes Lord Ebrington's remarks on the inspection of St. James's neighborhoods in 1845, particularly referring to the oft-cited

neighborhood of Golden Square, close behind the magnificent thoroughfare of Regent Street. It is a quarter inhabited by the most respectable of the labouring classes. These families for the most part have but one room, about twelve feet square, in which they sleep and live and some carry on their trade besides. . . . We did not see one healthy face. . . . Some of these rooms were over crowded cowhouses . . . the walls were filthy, the smells either abominable or exchanged for a closeness still more oppressive; the passages dark and tortuous. (15–16)

And yet the author emphasizes, "[H]ere were living the most respectable of the labouring classes." The author provides recent death rates in three areas in the parish: St. James Square (1 in 90) against the two problematic districts of Golden Square (1 in 36) and Berwick Street (1 in 42). These death rates are for 1845–1846, which were not years of particularly high mortality.

The author concludes that these "abominations [exist] . . . not in a parish like Spitalfields, but in one where Court is held, where palaces and palatial clubhouses and the mansions of the great [are located]" reminding his readers that

[t]he wealthy man in his mansion with its capacious rooms . . . is too apt to imagine that he is secure from the pestilential closeness of the densely populated and miserable neighborhoods which lie on the other side of him. But in that wretched locality, with which he would fain avoid all communication, and among the population so neglected, the seeds of disease are for ever rooting themselves afresh. (19)

Lest this pious warning fall on deaf ears, however, he points to another danger:

It is not, however, merely the health of the rich. . . . Their property, so dear to them . . . is in more way than one endangered. The inevitable moral condition of a population, located as has been described, has been ably depicted in the Sanatory *[sic]* Reports. . . . What can be expected of those who grow up with every local incentive to evil . . . ? (20–21)

In 1848, these descriptions are reaffirmed by the rector of St. James's who cites, rather inarticulately, several locations as filthy and impoverished: these include Angel Court on King Street, Golden Square—"The filthy condition of this place is scarcely to be described" (Jackson 7); Marlborough Row, Smith's Court on Great Windmill Street—"It is scarcely possible adequately to describe this plague spot of the parish" (Jackson 8); Ham Yard on Great Windmill Street; Peter Street; Hopkins Street; and a few others. It is unlikely that this situation had changed very significantly by 1854, especially as we know that the residents of Golden Square were still compelled to use the Broad Street pump as their primary source of water. However, in the report of the St. James's Cholera Inquiry Committee on the epidemic, we find:

Character of the Population—Confining our attention now to the district particularly affected . . . the great mass of the persons inhabiting the densely crowded parts is composed of the families of labourers, mechanics, and journeymen (many of them tailors), of persons, in short, employed at fair wages and manifesting no peculiarity in moral characters, habits or occupation beyond those usual to their class.

The author explains further in a footnote:

It was found, in the epidemic of 1849, that through London generally there were fewer deaths from Cholera on Wednesdays, Thursdays and Fridays. . . . The highest mortality took place on Mondays and Tuesdays. This difference was attributed in part to the indulgences often practised at the beginning and ending of each week. In St. James's, however, the greatest number of attacks was on Friday, and the daily range of mortality does not justify any general inference unfavorable to the habits of those who were seized,—a conclusion entirely in accordance with their varied position in society, and also with the assertions of those who know the district.

It is significant that although this report mentions the moral and economic habits of the people living in the densely populated areas, it says nothing about their sanitary condition! Yet, some description of sanitation would normally quite naturally have been included in such a report. For these inspectors, sanitary condition is conflated with economics and therefore morality: these tailors are employed regularly, and are temperate in their habits; therefore, they are cleanly. Even more importantly, though, they are conflated with and read through the lens of place. Many of the deaths in St. Giles were of respectable working-class people, yet they were shrugged off as "poor people" suffering the inevitable consequences of their lifestyles, which included location. St. James's poor, however, were emphatically to be read as respectable, and their deaths must be accounted for by other means. Clearly, just as St. Giles parish included many streets with respectable tradespeople and even middle-class families living in comparative cleanliness, comfort, and wealth, St. James's included many impoverished persons living under the worst of conditions.

In fact, the parliamentary report concludes that there is no reason to believe Snow's report, and that the death rates in St. James's are entirely consistent with existing theories: "[T]hat such local uncleanliness prevailed most intensely throughout the suffering districts is evident from the reported results of house to house visitation. . . . [T]he inhabitants were overcrowded, perhaps to the greatest degree known even in London" (*Report of the Committee for Scientific Inquiries* 51). 1851 statistics on population density, often cited as a measure of healthiness (moral and physical) in this period, bear this out: the population of Berwick St. was 1,524 people in 102 houses ("Supplement" 111). In terms of number of persons per acre, St. James's slums are worse than St. Giles. The populations of the three districts of St. Giles which had cholera deaths are as follows: St. George, Bloomsbury, 138 per acre; St. Giles, North, 291 per acre and St. Giles, South, 317 per acre. Compare these figures with St. James's hard hit areas: Golden Square, 166 per acre; St. James Square, 212 per acre; and Berwick Street an astonishing 432 people per acre. Yet although these truths were acknowledged within the parish by the officials who administered these areas, the image evoked by the proper noun "St. James's" was in no way tarnished by these facts, nor was "St. Giles" redeemed thereby.

Indeed, in 1850, Beames, who was a preacher and assistant at St. James's, Westminster, had called attention to Berwick St. (and Pye Street, Westminster) as well as St. Giles's in his *Rookeries of London*. He opens the chapter on St. Giles with this observation:

> We have stated that the most aristocratic streets have a background of
> wretchedness,—this at first sight seems incredible. We are too apt to suppose
> that St. Giles's is the only very poor quarter in London . . . [but] the better
> class of artisans and policemen are much straitened because of the dearness

of lodgings; the places where they live are destitute of most of the comforts and some of the necessary conveniences of life. Still we do not term their dwellings Rookeries, yet . . . few parishes are without . . . tenements which it would be difficult to describe by any other name. As a sample of this, let us survey part of the Berwick Street district of St. James, Westminster. (106)

We find, however, that despite the careful assertion that these are the "better class of artisans and policemen," once we arrive at the site in question, the inhabitants become "sweeps and costermongers, the usual number of idlers lounging about . . . suspicious looking characters . . . Irish, the vernacular language" (110). This does not seem to tally with other sources' (or even, as we have seen, Beames's own) description of the Berwick Street population; it is difficult to tell whether other sources have failed to recognize this class out of its presumed natural habitat, or whether these are actually respectable working tailors and the like and Beames can only define poor slum dwellers as Irish costermongers, or thinks his readers can. He continues to define the locals as thieves and drunken brawlers and notes darkly, "Inquests are common in this locality—many persons die by violence" (113). Despite Beames's helpful and very full description, however, he appears to have been quite right about the propensity of the general population to resist belief in very poor neighbourhoods outside of St. Giles.

The point here is not that there weren't real differences between the slums of St. Giles and those of St. James's; there were, and there were many good reasons that the Rookery should have been selected early on for demolition while Berwick Street remained untouched. St. Giles harbored many criminals, and the Rookery was a good geographic candidate for elimination as part of the New Oxford Street extension. But in sanitary terms, there were fewer differences. Given the reports of sanitary inspectors of St. James's, it should have surprised no one, believing as most did that cholera was caused by dirt and noxious odors, when Golden Square and its environs (especially Berwick Street) suffered "upwards of five hundred fatal attacks of cholera in ten days" in 1854, in "the most terrible outbreak of cholera which ever occurred in this kingdom. . . . The mortality in this limited area probably equals any that was ever caused in this country, even by the plague" (Snow, *On the Mode* 38).

Certainly it was far worse than had occurred in St. Giles that year. Whereas in 1849 St. Giles suffered 285 deaths from cholera, or 53 in 10,000 (according to Snow's tables, 62), St. James's had suffered only 57 deaths, or 16 in 10,000. St. James's deaths in 1854 totaled roughly 616, according to Snow's figures, 497 according to Parliamentary investigation, whereas St. Giles totaled 115 ("Supplement" 111). However, even before this devastating attack, traced by Dr. Snow, famously, to the contamination of the Broad Street pump by sewage, St. James's was suffering heavier mortality than St. Giles. In 1853, when the disease first began to be epidemic in London, St. James's suffered 9 cholera deaths to St. Giles's 1, or 25 in 100,000 to 2 in 100,000 (Snow 71). In fact, Snow's numbers show that the Western districts generally suffered mortality rates which exceeded those of the East and in fact, out of all districts, were only themselves exceeded by the death rates in the south: for example, Southwark, Rotherhithe, and so on (*On the Mode* 88). Snow further notes of the St. James's deaths:

> The limited district in which this outbreak of cholera occurred, contains a great variety in the quality of streets and houses; Poland Street and Great Pulteney Street consisting in a great measure of private houses occupied by one family, whilst Husband Street and Peter Street are occupied chiefly by the poor Irish. The remaining streets are intermediate in point of respectability. The mortality appears to have fallen pretty equally amongst all classes, in proportion to their numbers. . . . [J]udging from my own observation, I consider that out of rather more than six hundred deaths, there were about one hundred in the families of tradesmen. . . . [T]wo hundred and six persons were buried at the expense of St. James's parish; this latter number includes many who died in the hospitals, and a great number who were far from being paupers [but their friends, who would have buried them, did not know, or were overwhelmed by problems of their own]. . . . The greatest portion of the persons who died were tailors and other operatives. . . . They were living chiefly in rooms which they rented by the week. (*On the Mode* 48)

Without taking Charles Kingsley's *Alton Locke* as an incontrovertible statement about the living conditions of all tailors, we can refer to the earlier reports on the sanitary conditions of these dwellings to infer that many of these tailors were living hand to mouth—if they are tailors and not Beames's costermongers. It is possible that Snow is being somewhat disingenuous here—perhaps if only the poverty stricken died, it would be much harder to interest readers in his explanation of the cholera's epidemiology. Certainly, looking at his map, it does not seem that the deaths were "evenly distributed" through all classes, and earlier he mentions that the mortality was probably very much curtailed by the removal of many families who fled the district. We may assume that wealthier families were more likely to avail themselves of this option than poor ones. It is ironic that the facts in the case of the St. James's epidemic would have supported the widely accepted, though incorrect, assumptions about the cause of the disease at least as well as the facts about any of the preceding epidemics in most urban locations in the kingdom would have supported it. However, in this case, mistaken generalizations about the quality of life in St. James's proved a more durable mythic narrative than that of moral environmentalism and the cholera. Perhaps because of this, John Snow's correct surmises regarding the epidemiology of cholera were able to gain some purchase on the public imagination.

The pairing of a set of metropolitan extremes had become an essential element in representing London, both as a generalized example of an urban space in which such extremes would be contained and reconciled and as a specific classed and racialized representation of the extremes of Great Britain represented in the metropolis.[10] According to the facts, the deaths in St. James's should have reinforced existing prejudices about the disease; it is ironic that the disinclination to face those facts may have had something to do with the tentative acceptance of Snow's theory, which has long been narrated as a triumph of fact over prejudice—the modern narrative of progress. But the intersection between St. James's as a perceived space, resistant as that perception was, and Snow's mapping of it did much to promote the conception of space of medics which reflected liberal knowledges of the time: because of St. James's resistance to being represented in the simple terms of class difference within which sanitary representations were all too easily assimilated (that is, poor people were dirty, dirty people caused and suffered from epidemic diseases), it was easier for Snow to promote a specifically medical model of the vulnerable urban population and the cholera. This medical model, with its ruthless equivalences of all bodies and sites as equally vulnerable to a disease which made no class or moral distinctions brought perceptions of the city closer to the liberal ideal in two ways. First, as we have seen in chapter 3, it connected the previously isolated and distinctive parish with the urban social body as a whole, subject to the same laws and influences. Second, it took another step toward the standardization of space, geography, and bodies which the liberal ideal of transparency and universality required.

In other words, by ignoring the specific and factual slum conditions of St. James's which would have made the old sanitary moral environmentalism an adequate explanation for the epidemic, and instead using the generalized nonfactual perception of St. James's as wealthy, or at least respectable, Snow robbed the cholera narrative of its moral and class investments and placed it on a scientific footing which assumed an equality of bodies. This equality was essential to the liberal vision of the social body based on statistical knowledge which assumed an equivalency between units of measurement, that is, people. This is the same logic seen in Snow's water map, which stressed the equivalence of all physical conditions and bodies affected with the single exception of water supply (here, of course, this equivalence was supported by the facts, persons receiving different supplies often living on the same street and in the same circumstances).

Despite the sanitarians' efforts to realize a vision of equivalence, despite their vision of a city rendered universally salubrious through geographic remediation, the sanitary model partook too much of the old class and moral environmentalist assumptions to effectively body forth a truly liberal vision of progress, because it failed to take as given the (potential) universal equivalence of bodies as well as environment. These class investments, the assumption of essential difference related to class and its other manifestations—including, increasingly since the mid-Victorian period, race—continued to dog social mapping and liberal theory long after Snow, and they continue today. But Snow's work represented a decisive challenge, and is a good example of a trend in mapping which gains strength following this period.

Again ironically, this trend was toward the realization of the ideal of the sanitarians which they themselves had been unable to convincingly represent: a utopian metropole to be achieved through standardization of the environment. It did not include a more perfect adaptation to the given or natural environment, interestingly, for a discourse that justified itself with claims that humans naturally required light, clean air, and water, but a restructuring of the natural and built environment toward a more perfect realization of their ideal. Snow's observations about the contamination of water were easily folded into general sanitarian distrust of moisture and seepage—water, to be useful, needed to be contained. Wetlands, marshes, and riverbanks were all inherently unhealthy, and now they seemed also to represent the illness and contamination of human bodies and their wastes. The sanitary and medical ideal was popularized as not only light and airiness but dryness. As projects for the discipline of London's wetness such as the embankment of the Thames progressed—a project closely tied in the public mind to the mid-1850s epidemic—dampness, seepage, and the river were increasingly identified with not only disease but barbarism, the failure of the metropole to contain its wastes and to live up to the responsibilities of a civilized society. Civilization required land that was higher than the level of the water which supplied it, as dry as possible, airy, and cool, and England was to be transformed in this image. (How this image was shaped by and impacted visions of a land perceived as the opposite of this is a subject we shall take up in chapters 6 and 7.) The narration of progress as a process of containment was closely tied to the mid-Victorian bildungsroman; as we shall see in the next chapter, London came to embody both this vision of the possibilities of the liberal self and its pitfalls. Social mapping of London provided a template upon which such a subjectivity could be related to the body, both individual and social.

5

Medical Mapping, the Thames, and the Body in Dickens's *Our Mutual Friend*

> In these times of ours, though concerning the exact year there is
> no need to be precise, a boat of dirty and disreputable appearance,
> with two figures in it, floated on the Thames, between Southwark
> Bridge which is of iron and London Bridge which is of stone, as
> an autumn evening was closing in.
>
> —Dickens, *Our Mutual Friend*

IN THESE FIRST LINES of Dickens's *Our Mutual Friend*, all of the iconic elements important to the novel are present: the degraded man, the pure girl, the Thames, and most importantly, filth: a dirty boat on a "filthy" river (44), with, as Dickens's Mr. Mantalini would have described it, a "demd, damp, moist, unpleasant body" in tow. Although Dickens ostentatiously disregards precision as regards the year, he is extraordinarily precise as regards location on the Thames, and this is appropriate in a novel in which urban space—a detailed mapping of the city, its filth, and its main water supply—will be thematically central. Middle-class Victorians, of course, were particularly concerned with filth, and for good reason. Illnesses thought to be caused by inadequate sanitation were often referred to as "filth diseases," and nineteenth-century London was rife with them. Filth was rotten, decomposing waste, especially animal and human waste, and most especially feces.[1] As Peter Stallybrass and Allon White have argued, the nineteenth-century city is organized around the binaries of filth/cleanliness and the constant fear of their transgression, or contamination, resultant from desire (136). This fear "was articulated above all through the 'body' of the city," which had to be surveyed to be controlled (Stallybrass and White 125–26).

By the midcentury, this surveillance, equated with the very essence of civilization, was institutionalized in the mechanisms of sanitary inspection and had entered both literary and visual culture, the latter principally in the form of sanitary maps. The sanitary movement responded to overcrowding and epidemic disease by emphasizing the dangers of filth. Accumulated waste that earlier had been perceived as an unpleasant but unavoidable reality of life in the city now seemed evidence of a vicious, even murderous, disregard for life. Bodily wastes were no longer simply by-products of the life process, but filth that would, given the chance, attack the body itself. The body's continence, which also marked the boundaries of the middle-class self, could only be preserved through a careful policing of the abject and the boundaries of the body. By midcentury, the "lower bodily strata" of the city were increasingly thematized as both disease and antimodernity. In turn, health and modernity came to be identified with containment of the city's and citydwellers' bodies.

We have seen some examples of how the city, as both site and actor, was narrated in popular and medical discourse during the cholera epidemics. But the city, as the symbol of modernity and the social body, as well as the icon of infection, disease, overcrowding, and so on, becomes an increasingly important literary symbol in this period as well. The confluence of epidemic disease, sanitary theory, and the development of medical mapping, arising from what was perceived as a specifically urban and modern crisis, led to new representations of the city as itself a body. In London, the work of John Snow on cholera and fecal water contamination focused public interest on the Thames, already long a topic of outcry because of its pollution, evident to both nose and eye. The city's dangers were represented by its filth. When cleanliness was next to godliness, London's filthiness seemed an index of national sinfulness and inadequacy. The city as body, defined by its central river, was also marked and marred by its polluted seepage. Civilization, light and clean, high and dry, was threatened by the dark, dirty lowlands bordering the oneiric river on which the city itself depended. Containing and managing the Thames became exemplary of the liberal project of self-containment that was essential to the success of the liberal state.

THE LEAKY BODY AND THE INCONTINENT SELF

Herbert Sussman has traced in detail Carlyle's use of images of liquidity and "pulpiness" to describe the unformed masculine self at midcentury, which only careful self-cultivation and control would enclose in a relatively firm and clearly defined structure. This structure was constantly threatened by the

atavistic and chaotic liquidity of the male psyche; without vigilant self-polic-
ing, Sussman suggests, the self was always in danger of dissolution. He traces
these anxieties specifically in Carlyle's musings on masculinity, but I would
like to suggest that this imagery was actually fairly pervasive in mid-Victorian
culture. Rather than (or in addition to) the raw and the cooked, one might
think of Victorian civilizational hierarchy as often being defined as the opposition between the liquid and the solid. Sanitary understandings of moisture
as disease producing were reinforced by Snow's observation that the reason
water was dangerous was that it was full of human waste. Cholera, a diarrhoeal
disease, literalized this undisciplined evacuation of fluids and linked it to the
uncontained human fluids associated with improper drainage, mapping the
individual body onto the built environment (and vice versa). But this was simply one powerful model of a more widely held understanding of the dangers
uncontrolled physicality held for the social body. Bourgeois individuality,
which was not exclusively masculine but certainly masculinized, was based on
a model of the body which contained and separated itself from the bodies of
others, but the sick, undisciplined body threatened to sink the individual, and
those around the individual, into the unreasoning mass of continuous,
embruted embodiment. The pulpiness within was always threatening to burst
the bounds of the skin, which defined, contained, and disciplined the individual. Just as, as Armstrong argues, combination is troped as sexual scandal in
the narratives of the midcentury, disruption in the social body is translated
into a lack of discipline, figured as a lack of bodily self-containment. In
women, this is indeed often figured as inappropriate sexual openness; in men,
it may be aligned with tropes of addiction and plotlines involving mass violence. But in either case, wetness and liquidity often ground descriptions of
the body disintegrating as a threat to the larger social body.

 These images are emerging in part out of a Galenic medical vision of the
body as dependent for its health on homeostasis and of illness as a deficit or
excess which unbalances that equilibrium. Bleeding, for example, might be
done by a medic to relieve the pressure caused by an excess of richness or volume of the blood. Thus, matter coming out of the body or going into it in a
manner other than the normal alimentary intake was itself, as Mary Douglas
defines filth, "matter out of place": such matter, though not itself necessarily
filthy, indicated a filthy or potentially filthy state within the body. By the mid-
Victorian period, this model of a body made vulnerable by its own instabili-
ties was being challenged by a model of a healthy body vulnerable to outside
filth, with most Victorian medics falling somewhere in the middle, claiming
that illness resulted from a precondition of instability within the body which
might be exacerbated by such proximate causes as sanitary nuisances and an
"epidemic constitution" of the environment.[2] Both epidemic and hereditary
disease were sites of anxiety, complicating the individualist model; one sees in

Bleak House that this is where Dickens is able to make his most telling points about social responsibility and interdependence. Still, the model of individual moderation and continence as a means of both self- and social control remained powerful, in both sanitary theory and political economy.

Dickens's 1850s and 1860s novels appeal to an iconography of leakage versus containment in the service of a notion of liberal individualism.[3] He employs traditional narratives of sexual openness (in women), greed, addiction and its psychological double, obsession, to indicate lack of self-containment. The character who succumbs to these dangers risks losing individual identity, becoming part of an undifferentiated and abject corporeal mass. Dickens uses the individual's struggle for bodily continence to stage the development of the disciplined, self-contained subject, and the clean, modern city. In *Bleak House,* the body that is "vicious," not self-contained, engenders in its own humors "the only death that can be died," spontaneous combustion, a death which ruptures and makes meaningless the boundaries of the body which should protect the subject's interiority, leaving a dripping, greasy effluvium (479). By the early 1850s, then, Dickens already had recourse to the leaky body to relate his treatment of sanitary reform to social responsibility. Between *Bleak House* and *Our Mutual Friend,* however, came an important change in the perception of London and its own "bodily fluids"—that is, its water supply.

MAPPING THE URBAN BODY

As we have seen, thematic mapping was an important tool for sanitarians which amplified existing spatialized models of social problems in this period. Before the significant use of graphic maps (which mapped not only disease, but also poverty, crime, religious practice, and educational access as the most common measures), written narratives described population attributes spatially, by parish, neighborhood, street, or house. London was a privileged site of such representations, to which Dickens himself largely contributed, in such publications as *Sketches by Boz,* as well as his novels and innumerable essays and occasional pieces. Victorian commentators as well as later ones tend to cast the city as a "monster," a huge "growth," a confusing profusion. A favorite narrative device was to rely on the initial representation of London as an unmanageable jumble and then to impose order upon it through hierarchical binaries used to contain the city's diversity. Often these would rely on well-known geographic symbols such as Tom and Jerry's move from upscale Almack's to the fictive All Max in the East End, or as we have seen, between St. James's and St. Giles.

Early sanitary maps also relied on a simple binary of clean versus filthy. Especially under the early sanitary movement of Chadwick, from the late

1840s through the mid-1850s, filth, carefully mapped onto the urban terrain preparatory to intervention, was an index of moral corruption on the body social and in the individual bodies which comprised it. Excise the filth from the urban and individual body, it was reasoned, and the health of the social body must follow. As the century wore on and gains were made in the most basic levels of sanitation, however, medical mapping began to suggest more sophisticated relationships between urban space and disease. Mapping such problems became more than a simple sanitary exercise of pinning-the-nuisance-on-the-city, and became an interpretive practice by which social experts elaborated theories of human behavior and the nature of modern society.

Statistical studies such as Farr's analyses of mortality and morbidity returns sought to standardize a basic human life trajectory and then grid the city based on variables which affected that standard in a given area—rates of fever, for example, or correlation between elevation and life expectancy. As Mary Poovey argues, such statistical studies sought to transform social space into an abstract space that would be homogenous and transparent. Densely massed populations of the poor and transient who eluded observation, or were perceived to, challenged that project of abstraction, a project intimately related to Britons' sense of their civilization's modernity. Maps comprised a dual project: the representation of a reality, which was, simultaneously, a disciplining of that reality. Sanitary maps sought to make transparent or visible the hidden and therefore intractable social or sanitary ills of the day, and representation itself performed a kind of containment, while providing a guide for reformers to achieving that clean, well-lighted translucency which was the ideal of sanitarians. Dickens both was fascinated by and largely contributed to shaping such representations, while remaining deeply suspect of what he saw as this project's utilitarian challenges to individuality.

MAPPING WATER QUALITY

As we have seen, the shift from a simple binary view of the city and sanitation to a more complex mapping coalesces around a dramatic moment in the history of epidemiology: Snow's mapping of the St. James's epidemic. Snow mapped, instead of visible filth whose dangers were easily understood by any layperson, a hidden relationship between filth and disease: the invisible subterranean pollution of a well by seepage from a nearby cesspool. The Broad Street well water had been visibly clean and tasted wonderful; Snow's analysis suggested that the reason it tasted so good was precisely the presence of contaminants which oxidized the water. Only an expert could tell what dangers lay hidden in the most innocent-looking features of the landscape. His maps, then, as opposed to sanitary maps which charted some visible, tangible object—say, a dungheap—as the source of disease, redefine urban space by the relationship of disease to hidden features of the cityscape. Whereas earlier sanitary writers had exhorted readers breathlessly to "go see for themselves" horrors that were "hidden" only because they were in out-of-the-way places, Snow drily and professionally observes that the real dangers are those that can't be seen.

Snow's second map (see fig. 3.2) doubled back to 1832 as Snow drew larger connections between water quality and disease. The water company map offered a new definition of a human community that went beyond a neighborhood or even a parish to encompass the entire population of the greater London area. These representations envision (and thus, in part, create) a larger spatial entity, which, although hitherto apparently comprised of discrete and unrelated monads, could now be understood as vitally connected and participating in the same structure. London, often described in this period as an organism loosely coterminous with the social organism of English society, could be defined, diagnosed, and displayed simultaneously in these documents as a massive entity, organized around the Thames. The human bodies, invisible on the map of homogenous space that is the city, are represented by the personification of the city itself as population. The monster finally, graphically, had an organic unity and a definite structure, organized around a circulatory system.

Sanitary mapping had long focused on water and drainage, and the filthy state of the Thames had long drawn commentary. In 1850, R. D. Grainger submitted as part of his appendix to the *Report of the General Board of Health* a "Cholera Map of the Metropolis 1849," with variable shading in blue ink, darkness correlated to severity of cholera outbreaks and, on a separate diagram, to elevation, which was exhibited in the registration districts (see fig. 5.1). He remarks, "By referring to the tinted map of London, which shows the more precise seat of the mortality in each district, the intimate relation existing between the activity of the disease and the proximity of the river will become still more apparent; the dark colour, which indicates the relative mortality, showing even at a distance, the general course of the Thames" (Grainger 33). The map itself is a rather remarkable statement, appearing at first to have been the victim of a spilt inkwell or a wandering Rorschach artist. In fact, the spreading dark blue inkstain, carefully blocked from coloring the river and then allowed to soak into the town around it more or less at will, captures both the meticulousness of such mapping and the impressionistic rendering of Londoners' fatalistic sense of uncontrollable spread. Now the additional possibility of underground seepage, as had happened under Broad Street, made almost any urban dampness suspect of being filthy. In short, midcentury medical mapping refocused public attention away from the isolated "nuisance" (though those were still important),

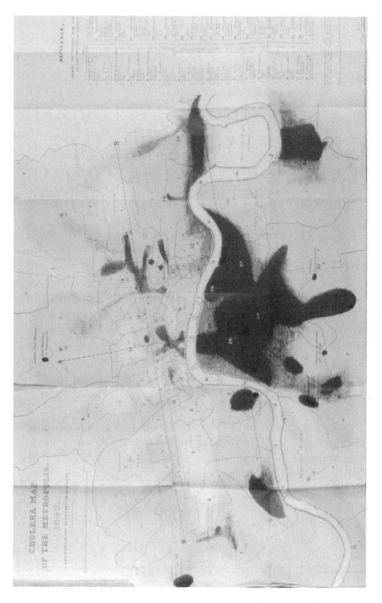

FIGURE 5.1. Grainger: "Cholera Map of the Metropolis 1849": detail. From Grainger, R.D. *Appendix B. Report of the General Board of Health on the Epidemic Cholera 1848 and 1849.* London: W. Clowes and Sons, 1850.

transforming the Thames into the primary site of London filth and a symbol of the dangers of uncontained fluids.

This shift in medical and sanitary understanding of water pollution took over a decade to fully penetrate popular understanding of disease, but its impact on those, like Dickens, who were *au fait* with the sanitary project, was immediate. The Thames in London is a tidal river: the daily tidal changes in the river's banks and the filthy residue of mud it left evidenced the river's tendency to carry the filth of the city's sewers back into the city itself, rather than away to sea. With the hypothesis of fecal-oral contamination, urban residents were forced to consider what had, in fact, long been obvious, if not as feared, that the water of the city traveled and retraveled through individual bodies from mouth to anus, just as the city's sewage flowed out to sea and back into Londoners' drinking cups with the tides.

LONDON'S BODY

The comparison between the novelist and the policeman or doctor as an expert in disciplinary diagnosis and surveillance has been ably explored by numerous critics following D. A. Miller. Let us simply say here that Dickens, like medical topographers, used what he considered his expert knowledge of both London and human nature to explore the hidden relationships between individuals who both constitute and threaten community. Dickens's work had long been part of the Victorian tradition of narrative topography and at mid-century, the influence of sanitary and medical maps gives his precise mapping of itineraries a new edge. Like medical mappers, he charts human actions onto the urban landscape and traces their hidden connections. As a sanitary activist, Dickens uses disease in *Bleak House* to show those connections; *Bleak House* is a medical map, doing exactly as other medical maps and sanitary narratives did to show how disease spreads from poor to wealthy neighborhoods, in the style of Kingsley's "Cheap Clothes and Nasty," or *Alton Locke*.

In *Our Mutual Friend*, following the paradigm shift set in motion by Snow, Dickens goes a step further. As Schwarzbach observes, Dickens "uses a language of social analysis and a model of social reform derived from the medical. . . . [T]he ideological structure of the text depends significantly on the discourse and paradigm of contemporary medicine" (93). But here, the disease becomes explicitly moral, rather than the actual fever which infects Esther, while the novel itself animates and narrativizes Snow's second map and subsequent investigations inspired by it—the medical mapping of fecal pollution of the Thames. No longer miasmatic, simply emanating from the slum Tom-All-Alone's, disease is no longer merely a symptom of social ills. Contagion didn't require the unlikely proximity of disparate populations that *Bleak House* did, because people didn't catch illness from other infected human bodies, but from the body of the sick city itself on which they depended symbiotically. Although Dickens retains the Galenic vision of a body whose fluids and solids must be homeostatically controlled—a vision which supports individual rather than community responsibility for continence—he combines this vision with one of a social body, mapped as London and its surroundings, whose vital fluid, the Thames, is contaminated as an index of the incontinence of London society. General physical incontinence, rather than specific disease, becomes the manifestation of a systemic social grotesqueness, and incontinence is persistently linked to the incontinent city's polluted water supply.

In *Bleak House*, the contaminated wetness of London breeds, miasmatically, disease and confusion, but we need not look to metaphor to understand that this moisture is filthy. Schwarzbach observes that "the mud [on Holborn Hill] is made up of dirt, rubbish (*dust* in English idiom), and raw sewage, ends up in the Thames and then oozes downstream to the Essex marshes. There it rots and festers, soon producing infectious effluvia that are blown by the raw East Wind back over the city. *This* is the stuff of the novel's dense fog . . . Dickens is pointing to a literal economy of filth and disease" (95). The scandal of filth in the heart of the modern city is an actual scandal, covered in the papers nearly daily, of the uncivilized, grotesque, leaky body persisting in the midst of civilization.

In *Our Mutual Friend*, the iconography of the individual and urban social body operates in much the same way as in *Bleak House*, although the connection between filth and literal disease is replaced by a more subtle portrayal of the body's vulnerabilities. Liquidity, garbage, filth, and waste constantly threaten the incautiously unselfcontained body, which must contain itself to build a financially independent, liberal self with a clear sense of identity.[4] Addiction—and greed for money comes under this heading in *Our Mutual Friend*—equates with desire for physical dissolution, for the abject. The unfortunate "Mr. Dolls," whose very name is unknown, drinks himself into a shambling and animalistic state of utter dependency; his body fails to hold together as he does finally "shake to bits" (714).

As in *Bleak House*, addiction can also manifest as obsession, either monetary or sexual. Eugene, the upper-class gentleman who appears to have the correctly contained bourgeois body but who lacks self-control, succumbs to a sexual obsession with Lizzie and a sadomasochistic obsession with Bradley Headstone (whose association with anality and anal rape has been elegantly elaborated by both Gallagher and Sedgwick). Eugene is beaten to a bloody and undifferentiated pulp and then dumped, like so much sewage, in the river from which Lizzie literally rebirths him (an act which finally rewards her own sexual self-containment, demonstrated by her mastery over the water, with middle-class status). Bradley Headstone himself is a man drowning in his own bodily fluids. He is unable to contain the blood which periodically spurts from his nose, causing fits: "I can't keep it back. . . . It has happened . . . I don't know how many times—since last night. I taste I, smell it, see it, it chokes me, and then it breaks out like this" (638). Unable to control the "wild energy" which has "heaved up" the "bottom of this raging sea" in his breast (396), appropriately, Headstone drowns. Incapable of governing his body, he pollutes the river with blood and the fluid excess of his desire; in turn, the polluted river invades his body and transforms it into the wholly abject.

Like the city which incontinently exudes and reabsorbs its own wastes, the incontinent body dissolves the boundaries of the self into the abject mass of physicality with which London's "dangerous classes" are associated, and with which Dickens (like other midcentury writers) connects barbarism. A male body which is inappropriately open to its own wastes or which, conversely, allows its vital fluid inappropriately to escape, represents a whole social economy in which individuals only distinguish themselves from the deathly mass of corruption by achieving a high and dry closure.

THE INCONTINENT CITY AND THE THAMES

Like the bodily economies of the individual characters above, London's economy is based on greed and fraud rather than continence—an inflated credit economy. The result of human incontinence is, according to the sanitarians, filth and results, at the social level, in a filthy city. Organized around the Thames, which gives the city both its structure and its connection to the outside world, medical mappings of London at midcentury, following Snow, began to portray the city as a system vulnerable through its polluted water sources. Dickens was preoccupied with the Thames even as he finished *Bleak House*. Concerned with the recent and returning cholera epidemic (1849 and 1854), he writes indignantly of those who would deny that contaminated water causes cholera (October 10, 1854, *Letters* 7: 435–36), and anathematizes "those Sewers Commissioners, who . . . really talk more rotten filth [. . .] than all the sewers of London contain" (7: 436). Dickens's concern with sanitary progress is of course well documented, and he locates Tom-All-Alone's in one of the hardest hit areas in the 1849 cholera epidemic (around the St. Giles area). In *Our Mutual Friend*, he is prescient; in the 1866 cholera epidemic, which was advancing toward Britain over the continent as *Our Mutual Friend* was being written, it was the docklands which suffered the worst mortality in the city on the north side of the river.

In this same letter, Dickens mentions George Godwin, editor of the *Builder*. Godwin's most famous popular works were two: *London Shadows* (on the homes of the poor, 1854), which Dickens read with interest, mentioning

Godwin on April 15, 1854, and October 10, 1854, in letters focused on homes and health (*Letters* 8: 313, 436), a topic with which *Bleak House* is intimately connected; and *Town Swamps and Social Bridges* (1859), which covers water pollution and sanitation at some length. Dickens corresponded with Godwin as late as November 30, 1865 (*Letters* 11: 116). *Town Swamps* was published in 1859, five years before Dickens began working on *Our Mutual Friend*. It connects Godwin's long-standing concern with sanitary housing with a discussion of water quality. The text includes several engravings, among which are one of an enormous dust mound in Nova-Scotia Gardens near Shoreditch (22), an area which was cleared under the direction of Burdett-Coutts, who knew both Dickens and Godwin well (see fig. 5.2).

While working on *Bleak House*, Dickens was heavily involved with Burdett-Coutts in her housing reform work, and it was Dickens who took Burdett-Coutts out to Nova-Scotia Gardens, the site of the giant mound depicted in Godwin's pamphlet. Godwin cites a "dense smell" associated with the mound, and the unhealthy condition of the neighboring tenements (23).[5] It is

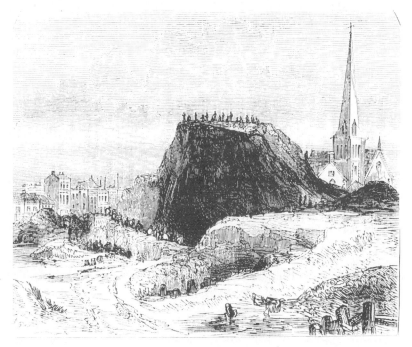

Nova Scotia Gardens, and what grew there.

FIGURE 5.2. Godwin: "Nova Scotia Gardens, and What Grew There." From Godwin, George. *Town Swamps and Social Bridges*. London: Routledge, Warnes, & Routledge, 1859.

possible that Dickens took his notion of the dust mounds from this connection, though there were certainly other mounds. In the same tract, Godwin emphasizes the tidal nature of the river and its effect on pollution: "[T]he sides and bottoms of boats become covered with solid matter; objects are not visible at even an inch below the surface" (56). He provides a sketch showing

> the way in which a dead dog, under our own eyes, traveled. We thought he would get away: however, after a time, and after whirling and resting amongst the posts and barges, the dead dog came again in sight, moving *against the tide,* but much nearer to the shore; he turns off again toward the sea this time much sooner than the last; and after describing various circles, as shown by the arrows in the sketch, he is deposited in the slime, together with other specimens of his and allied families. (56, emphasis in original; see fig. 5.3)

The water, which before Snow's work was popularly thought to sufficiently dilute and then wash the sewage out to sea, appears now as an invasive presence—moving, yes, but moving the same wastes into and out of the city repeatedly until its filth simply settles in place. My purpose here is not to suggest that the inspiration for *Our Mutual Friend* came from Godwin's pamphlet, though I think it quite likely that it made some contribution. Coverage of the water quality issue was of course widespread, and as a public figure interested in sanitation, Dickens would have seen most of this material. But given Dickens's pledge not to let the cholera issue die, or the water companies escape scrutiny, and given that cholera was again marching toward Britain as Dickens was writing, it is not surprising that the Thames and its purity would become an organizing metaphor for the problems of the city in *Our Mutual Friend.* The tidal nature of the river would become an important metaphor for the reverses and interdependences of the apparent social hierarchies of the city, and the plot would depend on an obsessive and recursive mapping of the river's course.

Bleak House used the Thames primarily as a setting for Esther's thematically crucial pursuit of Lady Dedlock, in which she loses her mother in order to find herself. As identity, the body and the city become central concerns in *Our Mutual Friend.* The novel, like London itself, is organized almost entirely around the Thames. It begins with an incontinent chapter of spills. Entitled "The Cup and the Lip," referring to balked plans as spilled drink, it begins on the river, between Southwark Bridge and London Bridge. Those whose plans are balked tend to land in the drink and are fished out by Gaffer Hexam, who is "allied to the bottom of the river rather than its surface, by reason of the slime and ooze with which" he, his daughter Lizzie, and his boat are covered (1). The bottom of the Thames is an abject place indeed, filled with sewage and decomposing flesh. We see Gaffer in the act of dragging up a body "in an advanced state of decay" (31).

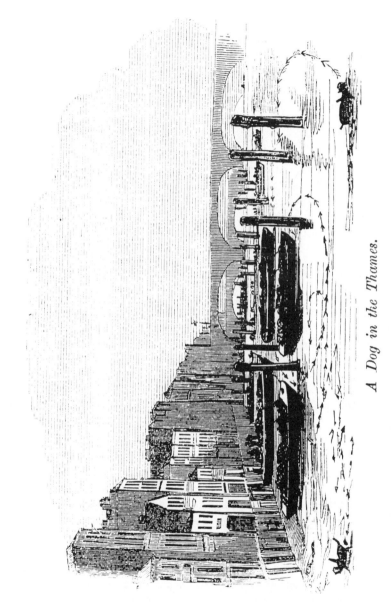

A Dog in the Thames.

FIGURE 5.3. Godwin: "A Dog in the Thames." From Godwin, George. *Town Swamps an Social Bridges*. London: Routledge, Warnes, & Routledge, 1859.

Poor Lizzie hates the river, even though it has been "meat and drink" to her; she resents being fed on dead bodies, and the river itself, at least in London, *is* a dead body, with a "sightless face" (5), much like the one Esther sees in the river on her hunt for her mother. Lizzie, like Esther, will undertake a quest for independence and freedom; for Lizzie, this will mean conquering the river, delivering it of life instead of death. Until she does so, she cannot leave its vicinity, although she wishes to. Her brother, escaping poverty into respectability, simply leaves the river and all the social rot it symbolizes far behind. When his sister tells him, "To please myself, I could not be too far from that river," he responds, mystified, "Why should you linger about it any more than I? I give it a wide berth" (228). But Lizzie knows she cannot win her independence by denying the social connection symbolized by the water source of London, and insists she must make "restitution . . . you know . . . Father's grave" (227) despite the fact that what she is making restitution for is not the actions of her father but the evils of society—the drowning of Jenny's drunken grandfather.

The river, then, represents something of what Tom-All-Alone's represents in *Bleak House:* disagreeable and dangerous filth emanating from the heart of the corrupt social domain of London which, however, cannot simply be ignored, because the social itself must be redeemed. If Gaffer Hexam, allied to the bottom of the river, is a degenerate father Thames, Lizzie will become the regenerating mother figure who will bring life out of the purer waters upriver. Like Esther, she will suffer for the sins of the world; like Esther, she will create the domesticity and love out of which redemption may emerge.

As in *Bleak House,* in which Chancery and "Fashion" are juxtaposed as mirroring oppositions in the first two chapters, *Our Mutual Friend* uses a similar technique in moving from the filthy river of the opening chapter to the society dinner at the Veneerings. Apparently opposite, the two scenes are actually similar, and Dickens will undertake to uncover these hidden correspondences. The dinner party is like the river, and Twemlow is a lost boat, trying to "take soundings" of an "abyss to which he could find no bottom." Much like the drinking water, this dinner is ministered to by a gloomy "Analytical Chemist" who is "always seeming to say, after 'Chablis, sir?'—'You wouldn't if you knew what it was made of'" and serves the dinner "as who should say, 'Come down and be poisoned ye unhappy children of men!'" (chap. 2). London society, meeting over its watery reflections in the Veneering table and plate, seems respectable and opulent, yet is rotten beneath the surface. Suitors deeply in debt court each other under the impression that there is wealth to be had, age masquerades as nubility, and Veneering's oldest and dearest friends scarcely know who he is. (In fact, though apparently very far from the filthy river, Veneering is a partner in a shipping firm.) Here we see the same opposition, then, as we see in the earlier novel: despite apparent differences, the social rot so evident at the docks begins here, at the heart of the apparently modern, clean city.

John Snow's report (and Godwin's pamphlet, quoting Snow) examines the role of the water companies in the 1849 and 1854 cholera epidemics, noting that whereas the Southwark and Vauxhall Water Company got its water at Battersea, heavily contaminated by sewage and subject to the incursion of sea water from the tide, Lambeth Water moved its supply in the early 1850s to Thames-Ditton. The result was, as Snow shows, that the two water companies supplied the same areas, but the customers of the Southward and Vauxhall company suffered initially over eight times the mortality rate of those supplied by Lambeth, and nearly five times the mortality in subsequent weeks. Snow asserts, "It is quite certain that the sea water cannot reach to Thames Ditton, any more than the contents of the London sewers" (Snow, *Snow on Cholera* 96). In fact, the normal dermarcation between the tidal Thames and the inland river is Teddington Lock, about two miles downriver of Thames Ditton:

> [T]he quantity of water which passes out to sea, with the ebb of every tide, is only equal to that which flows over Teddington Lock. . . . In hot dry weather this quantity is moreover greatly diminished by the evaporation taking place from the immense surface of water exposed between Richmond and Gravesend, so that the river becomes a kind of prolonged lake, the same water passing twice a day to and fro through London, and receiving the excrement of its two millions and more of inhabitants. (Snow, *Snow on Cholera* 95)

Shortly thereafter, however, John Simon observed, "Lower than Teddington Lock, indeed, the Thames may not be used as a source of supply; but above that point there dwell . . . very considerable urban populations" which may pose a hazard in the near future (Simon, *Report on the Last Two* 12). The use of Teddington as a line of demarcation between London and the country would increasingly come into question over the next decade.

In 1866, shortly after the final publication of *Our Mutual Friend*, cholera struck London. The areas hardest hit were those near where the river was most polluted—the East End dock area (see fig. 5.4), the area Dickens maps in *Our Mutual Friend* as the site of identity loss and construction. Dickens sets the first chapter in one of the Thames's most polluted areas somewhat further west, between Southwark Bridge and London Bridge. In a July 7, 1858, letter, he writes, "The Thames of London is most horrible. I have to cross Waterloo or London Bridge to get to the Railroad . . . and I can certify that the offensive smells . . . have been of a most head-and-stomach distracting nature. . . . [I]n the meantime, cartloads of chloride of lime are to shoot into the filthy stream, and do something—I hope" (*Letters* 8: 598).

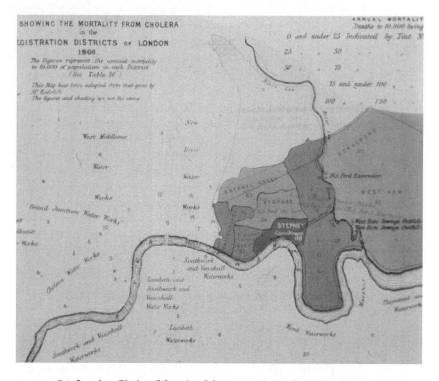

FIGURE 5.4. London Cholera Mortality Map, 1866: detail. From Farr William. *Report on the Cholera Epidemic of 1866 in England, supplement to the Twenty-Ninth Annual Report of the Registrar General.* London: George E. Eyre and William Spottiswoode, 1868.

Eugene masquerades as a lime merchant as a plausible cover for his presence at the docks. Dickens also pays careful attention to the sanitary condition of the river in placing his characters. For example, Riderhood suggests to Headstone that Eugene has lost the tide near "say Richmond" (632), thus stressing that they are at low tide and are therefore above the area in which the city affects the purity of the water. (Headstone will wait for the morning and the risen tide to follow.)

If Plashwater Weir Mill Lock is supposedly above the sewage of London and the tidal influences that can carry it, Greenwich is far enough east in the estuary that the ocean water dilutes and purifies. But this apparent purity is deceptive. In his mid-1850s work on cholera, Snow notes, "The great prevalence of cholera along the course of rivers has been well known. . . . Rivers always receive the refuse of those living on the banks, and they nearly always supply, at the same time, the drinking water of the community so situated. It has sometimes been objected . . . that the epidemic travels as often against the stream as with it. The reply to this is, that people travel as often against the stream as with it, and thus convey the malady" (*Snow on Cholera* 124). Eugene Wrayburn and Bradley Headstone carry the contagion of the city upriver to the purity of the rural areas there. The filthiest character of all, the Rogue, tends the lock in a lovely rural area which Dickens says "*looked* tranquil and pretty" (629, my emphasis). Dickens has Betty Higden live in Brentford: around the same time that the Lambeth company moved to Thames Ditton, the Grand Junction water company moved in the 1850s to obtain their water supply at Brentford, a few miles downstream of Teddington where they held it in a settling reservoir, thus cleaning it (65). Thus, "muddy Brentford" is a liminal point: not itself pure, it at least it does not produce poison, as any spot downriver would. Yet Johnny dies of a fever which is likely a filth disease.

The Lizzie-Eugene-Headstone plot moves further upriver to the west where the Thames upstream is initially associated with purity. Betty Higden, attempting to evade the Poor Law Guardians, takes "the upward course of the river Thames as her general track" where "you may hear the fall of the water over the weirs . . . and see the young river, dimpled like a child, play-fully gliding away among the trees, unpolluted by the defilements that lie in wait for it on its course" (504). Yet she is blackmailed by that very urban character, Riderhood, before she finally dies near the border of Oxfordshire (530), in the Upper Thames Valley. For Betty Higden, drowning is not a fate to fear but a mercy offered by a "tender river . . . the relieving Officer appointed by eternal ordinance" (504–5). Still pushed to "prove her independence" by her fear of the Parish, she falls prey to Riderhood, who robs her by threatening her with the relieving officer. She finally dies near the border of Oxfordshire (530), which suggests she is perhaps almost to Henley on Thames when she is found by Lizzie.[6] In 1865, the "Commissioners Appointed to Inquire into the Best Means of Preventing the Pollution of Rivers" were hearing evidence on the state of the upper Thames. One thing they were particularly interested in was the effect of the mills operating near Oxford, which used and polluted river water. In the Minutes of Evidence, lock keeper Mr. Bossom responds to a query asking if he is ever "troubled with refuse discharged from the University paper mill" by saying, "A lot of stuff comes from there. The stuff kills crawfish, and other fish as well. The stuff sometimes comes up black as ink" (*First Report* 2: 18). It is worth not-ing that Lizzie works in a mill just south of Oxford.

The condition of the river led to discussions of the connection between these small towns, with their local authorities, and London. M.P. Charles Neate notes that although the "original principle of the Thames Commission was to separate the fresh water river from the tidal river . . . at Teddington . . . no effective system of Thames management can be established without deal-ing with the mills" (*First Report* 2: 21). And Henry Acland, called in for his authority on cholera and Oxford geography, observed that "the river water above Oxford is fair enough. Below Oxford, for some distance, I believe it to be quite unfit for drinking" (*First Report* 2: 72).

Many of the respondents specifically identify the condition of the Thames as a national, rather than local affair, and interestingly, the reason given for this is generally its effect on the health of London. Acland stresses that he wouldn't consider the pollution of the Thames around Oxford a matter to be solved by local planning because "I am not only an Oxford man but an Englishman. . . . All our local purposes will be gained by joining in the amelioration of the whole" (*First Report* 2: 72). Another witness, Mr. Harrison, a lead merchant at Reading, insists that the "deplorable, filthy state" of the Thames is a matter of national importance "because the inhabitants of London and the whole of the Thames valley depend for their supply of water on the Thames" (*First Report* 2: 114). The apparent cleanliness of Dickens's rural river is meaningless; Headstone, fitting emblem for a rotting body, soils it with blood. In insisting on the deceptiveness of the river's apparent purity, Dickens stresses here the *Bleak House* lesson of connection between places and people apparently quite widely separated, of interdependence between city and suburb, but he uses Snow's connection of the river and pollution to do what a miasmatic model of disease and contagion from Tom-All-Alone's did in the earlier novel. Like Snow, he also emphasizes the opacity of those connections to the uninitiated eye—it is the novelist who can map the hidden contamination, while the reader must yield to his expert construction of the city's space.

Identity loss is of course a key theme of the novel, and most critics have noted how often that loss is tied to immersion in the river. It is important also to note that the novel identifies the interpenetration of city and river with this loss as well: individual identity loss is mirrored by the city's boundary diffusion. As Deirdre David notes, Dickens began writing *Our Mutual Friend* as the Thames was being embanked and efforts were being made to establish better drainage near the river in the East End (53; see Dickens's letter of November 30, 1865, *Letters* 11: 116). The novel, however, relies on the river's unembanked state, its pollution of the surrounding land and the uncertainty of its boundaries, to point to the porosity of the selves the principal characters are struggling to contain and define. As in *Bleak House*'s Tom-All-Alone's, social detritus is compared to human waste, and the Thames as both the organizing metaphor and landmark of the novel seems at key moments to incorporate the city along its banks: Rotherhithe is "where accumulated scum of humanity seemed to be washed from higher grounds, like so much moral sewage, and to be pausing until its own weight forced it over the bank and sunk it in the river . . . among vessels that seemed to have got ashore and houses that seemed to have got afloat" (21).

The loss of identity is associated with bodily transformations. In the above scene, Mortimer and Eugene go to the riverside to misidentify John Harmon's decaying body. When Riderhood goes in turn to misidentify Hexam as the murderer, he once again leads Eugene and Mortimer to the water, walking through hail in which his footprints leave "marks in the fast-melting slush that were mere shapeless holes; one might have fancied, following, that the very shape of humanity had departed from his feet. . . . [I]t seemed as if the streets were absorbed in the sky, and the night were all in the air" (157). Riderhood loses the boundaries of his body as the city loses its definition. But in this night of transformations it is Hexam's drowned corpse that will emerge from the river, after a long night in which Eugene impersonates a lime-merchant, Mortimer, in exhaustion, hallucinates, and Eugene himself feels that he is being transformed into a "half-drowned" criminal who has "swallowed half a gallon" of the "wash of the river" (164). On the river itself, "[E]verything so vaunted the spoiling influences of water—discoloured copper, rotten wood, honey-combed stone, green dank deposit—that the after consequences of being crushed, sucked under, and drawn down, looked as ugly to the imagination as the main event" (172). Worse, what goes into the river comes back out and is incorporated back into the city's bodies, as we are reminded in the first few pages of the novel by Gaffer, who responds to poor Lizzie's river aversion by insisting that it is "meat and drink" to her. In (and for) London, loss of identity also means abjection, the grotesque loss of the body's integrity.

Despite their many trips to the sea or the countryside, the principal characters must still go to this place and face the worst of the river to claim their true identities; that is, they must overcome the filth with which they are contaminated and for which they are in part responsible. The river, damaged as it is, represents potential redemption, as the main organizing principal and water source for London must (as many critics have discussed, most notably Deirdre David). Harmon loses his identity in his waterside adventure, but is also able to fashion a new and more secure self after his slow rebirth. On a night when the water of the river is blown through the air like the rain (365), setting up the river-city boundary blurring associated with identity loss, he attempts to reconstruct the night he lost himself, having been disguised and drugged: "[T]here was no such thing as I, within my knowledge" (369). Being thrown into the Thames in an attempt to finish him off paradoxically revives him, and he thinks "[T]his is John Harmon drowning! John Harmon, struggle for your life. John Harmon, call on heaven and save yourself!" . . . [Finally] it was I who was struggling alone in the water" (370). In this struggle to re-form and contain himself, to call himself into being, he confuses himself by actually crossing the river; he cannot reorient himself: "Even at this moment, I cannot conceive that [the river] rolls between me and that spot, or that the sea is where it is" (370). He is, as the narrator describes him, a "living dead man" (373), as if his soul has been left in hock to the underworld. He attributes some of his unease to the lingering effects of the drug: "[E]ven now, I have sometimes to think, constrain myself . . . or I could not say the words I want to say" (371). Retracing his steps and remapping his body's (and London's) location in relation to the river is part of the process of consolidating his new self.

The metaphors here are all of containment. Like the river, Harmon's subjectivity exceeds its boundaries; he must be "constrained," put back in his container, his body made fast against forces external to it—the drug, for example, or the water. In fact, as with Eugene and Lizzie, Harmon's long slow birthing out of the Thames cannot be finalized without Bella's love and marriage. It is not until after his marriage, the birth of his child, and the clearing away of the dust mounds that he is able to claim the name he calls out over the river. Not until Bella declares her faith in him and her innocence of any untoward desire for wealth does she too, in "the state of a dreamer" go to the "low-lying water-side wharves" near London Bridge (762) where all, down to the drunken woman banging on the cell door, is as it was when the body of "John Harmon" was found. Again, they go to the Six Jolly Fellowship Porters where, this time, John Harmon's living body will be correctly identified. And here, this time, Bella will lose her identity as Mrs. Rokesmith in order that both she and her husband may be reborn as their true selves, the Harmons. The project of embankment, providing definite boundaries between land and water and containing the pollution therein, matches the project of defining and defending clear boundaries of the self.[7]

Eugene's mutinous thoughts before the attack are compared to the rippling of the river as he walks beside it; they sweep him along on the current of his desires for Lizzie, and he seems to blend with the water as he stares into it (698). Again, this merging with the water signals a potential loss of self. Moments later, Headstone ruptures Eugene's body, paralyzing him and causing him to bleed nearly to death after he dumps him in the river. The face of the river which Lizzie earlier feared seeing is literalized when she sees "a bloody face turned up towards the moon" (699). "Insensible" and "mutilated," Eugene's body—described now simply as "it"—"streaked the water all around it with dark red" (699). As with John Harmon before him, Dickens carefully explains that Eugene crosses to the opposite side of the river from his inn, having gone there for the quiet, so that Lizzie must bring him across the river to save him. Not having emerged on his own, Eugene is even further than Harmon from achieving a reintegration, and for many days "no spirit of Eugene was in Eugene's crushed outer form" (736). He keeps "losing himself" in "endless places" at an "immense distance" (738). Though there are fleeting attempts to collect himself, any expression on Eugene's shattered face is "so evanescent it is like a shape made in water" (736). It is finally the effort to deflect public attention from Lizzie which enables him to focus, and his marriage to her that gives him strength to live. He declares his determination to go back and face London society.

The women of the novel, with the exception of Bella and Mrs. Lammle, are largely innocent of the sins for which the men must be purified through a "filthy" baptism. Helena Michie has identified both *Bleak House* and *Our Mutual Friend* as novels in which women's bodies are made to suffer scarring and disfigurement in order to constitute a self, yet, as Catherine Gallagher has pointed out, all the wounded, drowned, and decomposed bodies in *Our Mutual Friend* are male. Both critics attend to Dickens's undeniable tendency to mortify the flesh of his characters, either in the pursuit of selfhood or to mark its disintegration. I would suggest that the testing and creation of the self in these novels and, indeed, in many Victorian novels, is often symbolized through lesions of the flesh, and success is marked, specifically, through the ability of the body to overcome breaches in its self-sufficiency; however, men can incur lesions incurred on their own behalf, whereas women can only heal those resulting from the sins of others. Gallagher explores the way in which males often seem to have "extra" commodified bodies, and through being "rearticulated" in the manner of Mr. Venus, often can birth new selves, whereas women only have one chance; if they lose that closure, it can never be regained. However, as Michie points out, women's bodies bear more scars in the novels for the sins of others, as Esther does in *Bleak House,* and as Jenny's body perhaps bears the sins of her drunken progenitors in *Our Mutual Friend.*

Lizzie and Betty Higden are already self-contained, unpolluted by their association with the river. Still, as in *Bleak House,* they suffer the results of others' incontinence. Lizzie herself sees her battle against her love and flight from Eugene as being quite similar to Betty Higden's battle to remain economically independent and flight from the parish; inspired by Betty, she says she is willing to die to preserve her self-respect. Still, she nearly loses—her heart had been "so full, and he the cause of its overflowing. . . . [S]he tried hard to retain her firmness, but she saw it melting away. . . . In the moment of its dissolution . . . she dropped" (694). Unable, for the moment, to support herself, dissolving into fluids by the riverside, she makes good on her promise of a moment earlier: "He held her, almost as if she were sanctified to him by death, and kissed her once, almost as he might have kissed the dead" (695–96). Her weakness calls out a reciprocal flow: Eugene covers his face to think, and is surprised to find that there are "tears in his hand" (696). Moments later, his bodily integrity will be much more severely compromised, and Lizzie will suffer with him, becoming completely unconscious once she gets medical help for Eugene. Like Esther crossing her "dark lake" to conclude her illness, Lizzie will carry her burden "back against the stream" and the voyage of self-realization which began amid the docks will be fulfilled, as it is in *Bleak House,* with marriage to a suitable, waterproofed man.[8]

WHOSE BODY MATTERS

We can see a clear continuity between *Bleak House* and *Our Mutual Friend* in terms of the sanitary rhetoric of the two novels. If *Bleak House* concerns itself more directly with contagious disease and the corruption of the home (as the title suggests), with the rupture between private and public, inside and outside, and therefore with the permeability of the characters' skin, *Our Mutual Friend* simply bypasses the public realm and follows social illness to the most basic font of the grotesque body, to the contamination of the city's body with its most abject waste—feces and rotting corpses. If *Bleak House* celebrates the individual's transcendence of social determinants even while it emphasizes the body's embeddedness in a community of contagion, *Our Mutual Friend* emphasizes individualism still more. The grotesque body is not made so by its connectedness to other bodies, as in *Bleak House*, but by its lack of self-control, just as the city is made grotesque through this same lack of planning and authority. Bradley Headstone lacks not opportunities for bourgeois selfhood, but the ability to contain himself. Betty Higden, on the other hand, though she dies outdoors, is self-contained and self-sufficient to the last, both financially and physically. Poor as she is, she emphasizes, she "paid scot and . . . lot . . . worked when she could . . . starved when she must" (200). Dickens is, of course, emphasizing the cruelty of making such a person feel pauperized by relief when she is starving, but he does so by playing into stereotypes of bourgeois self-sufficiency. Picking up on the current Reform Bill debates about the fitness of property renters and owners, he indicates that she paid the property taxes (scot and lot) which would have made her potentially fit for the vote were she a man. Dickens underscores this with reference to her physical self-control; when crying for the potential loss of Johnny, "the fine strong old face broke up into weakness and tears" (202), but then she declares her independence of the parish, and "there was no more breaking up of the strong old face into weakness. My Lords and gentlemen and Honorable Boards, it really was as composed as our own faces, and almost as dignified" (204).

The weak, like Headstone and Eugene, disintegrate; the strong do not "break up," but "compose" their bodies, as the dying Betty does when she arranges herself under a tree next to her "orderly" basket and carefully places her letter on her dying body where it will be seen, so she will not be buried by the parish. As Sloppy eulogizes her, "She went through with whatever duty she had to do. . . . [S]he went through with herself, she went through with everything" (516). This is the individual as project with a vengeance, and Lizzie and even Jenny, crippled but not grotesque, must follow this model of industrious self-construction, as do John and Eugene.

We have already observed that women's bodies mediate identity and closure differently from men's, and it is important to note that men's bodies and subject formation differ along class lines in the novel. Unlike the upper class men whose identities are sufficiently protean that the dip in the river helps them to consolidate a self, Headstone's self is too essential and too much with him. He spends plenty of time in the river, but is uncleansed. His final ordeal by water begins when Riderhood appears in his classroom and asks the children, "Wot sorts of water is there on the land?" "Seas, rivers, lakes and ponds" is the chorused response. (794). He does this to remind Headstone of the identity—his own—which Headstone tried to steal by disguising himself and then sinking the clothing in a pond. But Headstone himself, that raging sea, is also water on the land and must return, finally, to his own element. Headstone looks both up and down the river he has defiled as Riderhood threatens to "drain him all the drier" for his delays. Then he drags Riderhood down into the "ooze and scum" at the bottom of the lock, where they will both be found dead. Riderhood imagines himself to be immune to drowning, as he too has been "drowned" before. But he hasn't crossed the river, as have Harmon and Eugene; he has failed to be reborn as self-sufficient and therefore he remains parasitic, a bloodsucker drawn to the blood which Headstone is unable to contain and which periodically spurts from his nose, causing fits: "I can't keep it back. . . . It has happened . . . I don't know how many times— since last night. I taste I, smell it, see it, it chokes me, and then it breaks out like this" (638). A man drowning in his own fluids, Headstone's own bodily incontinence, which begins as he hunts Eugene, leads him to draw the blood of another. As Bradley imitates Riderhood, he becomes not less, but more like himself (631), so tenuous was the respectable, contained self he had created. Paradoxically, the only way he can redeem coherent selfhood or control over his own body is through the final destruction of the irreparably ruptured creature he has become.

Again, it is a woman who saves him; it is his desire to spare Miss Peecher that decides him to take the step he has been thinking of since before his attack on Eugene. Stalked by Riderhood as he himself stalked Eugene, he does what Eugene was unable to do when he tried "dragging at his assailant" (698): he pulls Riderhood into the water with him. The two kindred natures become one in death in a lovers' embrace, and in this way Headstone asserts the unaltered, classed core identity which his performance of a middle-class, self-contained self, maintained with so much costly effort, obscured. These class differences mark the fact that, despite Dickens's use of similar themes in the two novels, and the greater elaboration of a notion of identity and the body which initially appears to be mapped onto the sanitary redemption of the city, *Our Mutual Friend* is, finally, as many critics have noted, a less socially critical book than *Bleak House.* Outside of the pointed critique of the Poor Law, Dickens contents himself with general admonishments to good behavior in sanitary terms. He offers little hope for the increased fitness of the working class through culture and education, as his contemporaries were doing during the long debates over the second Reform Bill; indeed, both Charlie Hexam and Bradley Headstone are clear examples that education and culture, at least when seen as a means for fulfilling ambition, neither morally ennoble those who acquire it nor overcome a core, classed self. He defends the amusements of the poor, as he has in *Hard Times,* against the critique of liberal contemporaries who would seek to elevate the tastes of the working classes (690), though Lizzie, of course, has no such working-class tastes. But he also portrays those amusements as pitiable and decrepit, offering "despairing gingerbread, that . . . had cast a quantity of dust on its head in mortification" (599–600). Given the associations of "dust" in this novel, such a spectacle is particularly unappealing.

In the case of Headstone, Dickens repeatedly hints that the pauper boy would have been better off had he embraced his destiny as a laborer, rather than repressing his true nature. In short, although the self-as-project is an important theme in the novel, the privilege of an active creation of the self is really restricted to the middle-class man such as Eugene or John. In *Our Mutual Friend,* franchise reformers' great slogan of liberal hope in the transforming powers of education on the working classes, "The schoolmaster's abroad," is stated with chilling effect by Eugene to a horrified Mortimer (541) as he describes leading his stalker over the entire topography of the city, especially through areas noted for their sanitary and social horrors such as Bethnal Green. Liberals agitating for voting privileges for skilled laborers tended to embrace a rhetoric of self-development: through education and careful self-management, workers could build middle-class subjectivity and demonstrate the bourgeois values that would prove their fitness as citizens. Certainly there are problems with this narrative, but this was still the dominant narrative among liberals. Dickens's message however, is quite clear. Though Eugene and John can be reborn out of the Thames, Riderhood, Headstone, and even the relatively innocent Radfoot and Hexam end their lives at the polluted bottom of the river.

This class disparity brings us back to Gallagher's argument that the illth/wealth distinction cycles through bodies as commodities; bodies must be used up in order to be recycled and renewed as wealth, and that only males have commodity bodies that can survive such recycling. She argues that the gender split emerges from both the feminine tendency to be naturally commodified and the feminine need to be saved from such commodification by males. Her reading is compelling; I would like to extend its implication to account for class difference between men in the novel, an issue Gallagher does not discuss. Strikingly, there is no class difference between women, as we have seen, and perhaps this is precisely because all the women of the novel resist commodification and are removed from this threat safely into domesticity by the novel's end. But if the middle-class males are able to exhaust themselves as commodities and then regenerate, recycled out of the filth and garbage into health and wealth, the working-class males who take on any real protagonism within the novel (as opposed to Sloppy or Boffin, who do not really develop from the static self-containment with which they begin the story) are doomed to failure. Any imbalance within their bodies results in filth, and only in filth, never in its reclamation.

Matter out of place, elevated beyond their own station, as Wegg and Headstone are, they can only leak, decay, and end at the bottom of the river or on the scavenger's cart. Even Boffin follows this trajectory, though it is all show; perhaps it can be all show precisely because the real heir has turned up and saved him from the fate of the miser which he enacts, to end as Dancer did, in a filthy dungheap. Instead, Sloppy and Boffin remain grateful to be comfortable within their own class and enjoy a limited social mobility within which they acknowledge the social superiority of the Harmons. Only bourgeois males can use up bodies and survive in this economy, and they can use up not only their own, but the bodies of others—a disturbing echo of a real economy of corporeal usage and wastage supporting a liberal subject who, like Esther, is as "innocent of its birth as a Queen" and whose containment acknowledges no debt to the vulnerabilities of others. It is Dickens's ambiguous endorsement of this closed self which makes his harsh judgment of Charley Hexam, who seems precisely such a self, suspect. He insists simultaneously that the successful self embank its metaphorical polluted river and implies that somehow the real river will likewise be embanked without showing that the successful self has any responsibility for doing so.

On the other hand, unlike *Bleak House,* there is no exodus, either to Yorkshire or other garden spots. Eugene considers the colonies, yet wants to face London society with Lizzie. The characters must continuously traverse the filthy, polluted urban stretch of the river, and all must pass the test of immersion near the docks to survive. Rather than tackling specific institutions in *Our Mutual Friend* (always excepting the Poor Law), Dickens responds to *Bleak House*'s diagnosis of a sick social body through the turn to individual self-containment. In *Bleak House,* lack of self-containment results in harm through poor sanitation which is caused by systemic corruption. In *Our Mutual Friend* the systemic corruption practically vanishes from the text except for parenthetic reminders; instead individual incontinence is mapped directly on to the body of the city without the mediation of a sick government or society at large.

If *Our Mutual Friend* is disorienting, it is because of this Gothic interiority in which each character seems isolated from a working society, not because of spatial vagueness. Dickens's mapping of the characters onto the city is precise. But the polluted cityscape comes to represent the incontinence of the characters' selves in their dangerous abjection. The entropic city faithfully maps subjectivity out of control, the flooding, filthy river bodies forth the desires that erode the boundaries of the embodied middle-class self. The embankment, after all, is a hopeful project, and in recommending the cultivation of a private, individualized self which finds its fullest expression in domesticity and economic self-sufficiency, Dickens is clearly hopeful that a society of such monads will modernize the city, eliminating the primeval mud and incontinent filth of barbarity. But the bodies that matter are those of middle-class males. Reform, with its rhetoric of liberal individualism, continence, and the self-as-project as models available to all, has no place on Dickens's map of London.

DICKENS, THE MONSTER, AND THE CRITICS

Much has been made of the chaotic nature of Dickens's urbanism in the later novels. Julian Wolfreys has argued that London is given to us as a "discourse always reshaping itself, emerging . . . as a monster" which cannot be fixed but leads us on through our desire, precisely, to "fix it in place, hold it in the gaze forever" (67). Citing Connor's work on both *Bleak House* and *Our Mutual Friend*, he refers to the long critical tradition of seeing in these texts a lack of specificity—or so much specificity that meaning evaporates, exposing the random nature of the city. Kay Hetherly Wright finds the key to *Bleak House*'s urban chaos in the grotesque, whereas Allan Pritchard seeks an understandable structure to *Bleak House*'s London in the Gothic. All of these readings attempt to account for the pervasive sense of disorientation in *Bleak House* and *Our Mutual Friend* in terms of a lack of realistic specificity, or at least a turn to a mode of representation other than realism.

In fact, however, the novels are quite specific—even fussily, journalistically so—about locations. I would suggest, following Wright, that the grotesque is indeed the structuring mode of these novels, and it is that which makes them seem dreamlike and unrealistic in its portrayal of space. But Dickens was portraying, through this mode, a very concrete set of conditions in London which he and his contemporaries perceived as both quotidian and monstrous or Gothic—the simultaneous existence of different temporal modes in the same space: the barbarism of the slum, the premodernity of the dredgers (who even shadow the triumphant moment of Bella's wedding as the mud-larks to whom her father declaims his wedding speech), and the physical presence of human filth in the very heart of the city, its contaminated river, which was persistently characterized as a barbaric stain on the civilized city in sanitary journalism. The timelessness of the Indian landscape we will see in chapter 6 erupts, through the uncontained body, into the temporal palimpsest of Western modernity. Thus, it is the body which is always potentially grotesque in these novels, and the mark of its grotesqueness is waste: excrement, blood, decaying corpses; the city is the material manifestation of the sick social body, and thus, must be grotesque as well.

Franco Moretti's brilliant mapping of Dickens's novel makes the important point that Dickens, over the course of his lifetime production, mediates the binary of East and West Ends by producing and populating a third space, that of the middle class, occupying the wedge of London including the City, the Inns and the suburbs north of those points between the corrupt West End of the aristocracy and the criminal East. It is a fine and compelling argument, though, as Moretti admits, not completely consistent. For example, Tom-All-Alone's in Bleak House sits as uncompromisingly in the middle of Holborn as St. Giles did, and many of Dickens's decent middle class are quite horrifying—Vholes, for example (and he, like many middle-class characters, is a suburbanite). However Dickens does indeed populate this pie piece of London with the middle class (as it actually was) and does indeed make that class his hero.

That said, it is important to pay attention to his characters' extraordinarily peripatetic tendencies. In locating their homes, Dickens indeed tells us a great deal about the characters' social position and so forth in a kind of shorthand. But the characters are very often not where they are supposed to be. True, the first chapter begins with socially marginal characters from the docklands. But they begin the novel between London Bridge and Southwark Bridge—by the City that Moretti identifies as middle-class space. As we have seen, one of the most shocking revelations of the 1855 epidemic and Snow's mapping of it was that the single worst local epidemic of this "filth" disease, so identified with poverty and immorality, happened in St. James's, while St. Giles, its abject opposite, was practically untouched. In fact, although many were shocked by the disease striking such an opulent and fashionable West End parish, no one should have been—Berwick Street near Golden Square was one of the worst slums in town, as we have seen. However, as Lefebvre points out, there is often a disjunction between perceived, conceived, and lived social space—that is, space as it understood to be, space as it is ideally planned to be by experts, and space as it is actually practiced by human beings. Except for the few people who lived in that slum, the social understanding of Golden Square by most Londoners was assimilated to its general location in a wealthy parish; Londoners thought that if people in St. James's could die of cholera, it could happen anywhere—the binary of filthy and clean, poor and rich had collapsed. Snow took advantage of this perception, dwelling on the respectability of the artisans who lived there rather than on their filthy and impoverished living conditions which would have fueled sanitarian rebuttals to his radical fecal-oral theory. In this way, perceived space tends to elide some of the complexity of lived space, just as the broad homogenizing tendencies of pitting East and West against each other, or even East, West, and Middle tend to do.

Dickens, then, both employs these binary oppositions and resists them in the interest of particularization. One of his abiding interests is the heterogeneity of local spaces, the surprise that is just around the next corner. To this end, he places characters' homes in locations which take advantage of readers' perceived-space mappings of London and then, like Snow's report, proceeds to demolish those boundaries as he shows just how vulnerable and porous they are to seepage.

As in medical maps, the binaries of the first half of the century give way in this novel to a more complex set of spatial relations. Plot interest, as Moretti points out, is often generated by the transgression of boundaries, and certainly some of the disorientation critics complain of is less a result of the novel's atopicality than of the difficulty of reconciling Dickens's meticulous detailing of transgressive itineraries with the binaries of Victorian London as perceived space. Like Snow, Dickens makes a point about the difference between perceived and lived space; like Snow, he both takes advantage of popular perceptions and challenges them, showing those mythic boundaries are meaningless in the face of the city's inability to maintain bodily hierarchies. If the West End with its palaces of government is the head and mouth of the city, the upper bodily strata taking in sustenance from the healthy countryside, and the East End is the cloaca, discharging toward the sea (and the Continent) the city's wastes, what does it mean that the corpse of George Radfoot dumped into the water in Limehouse Hole washes up in the City? Partially, of course, Dickens wants the association of filth with the financial and market districts—the body is hauled up right by London Bridge—to tie the waste-wealth equation together. But this is possible because the tidal river invades east to west, an inversion of bodily and imperial hierarchies, just as the cholera both globally and locally associated with the East appears in St. James's to the horror of both the wealthy and the middle class.

Dickens's project, then, much like the sanitary mapping project, was to abolish the perceived mythic spaces of London—that is, a London of tightly contained and class-distinct areas—in favor of a realist understanding of London as a lived space of heterogeneity and conflict. This demystification is not simply celebratory, however; it is a preparatory step to bringing London into line with the conceived space of mappers and medics—in this case, an idealized vision of the London in which the disorder which disrupts boundaries is abolished and all areas become homogenously bourgeois. The dominance of middle-class space which, as Moretti demonstrates, emerges in this text is thus as much utopian inner space as actual geography. Order cannot be imposed simply by cordoning off the "dangerous classes"—they just jump in a boat and row west—but by transforming them, whenever possible, into continent individuals.[9]

Snow and his contemporaries transformed the cholera from a moral issue into an engineering problem—one not of prayer or temperance, but simple physical containment. As we saw in earlier chapters, the project of urban transformation was finally as much a psychogeographic one as one of actual rebuilding, yet this project was ultimately depoliticized even as it became more firmly rooted in liberal thought, because it was increasingly individualized. The sanitary project of purifying the water supply and the city through careful containment become the emblem of a society's attempt to civilize itself through the containment of its constituent bodies and the reshaping of individual selves, leaving Dickens and his readers gazing, with cautious optimism, at the new Thames Embankment.

PART IV

Mapping the Body of Empire

6

India in the 1830s

Mapping from the Professional Periphery

> The men who won an empire, and stood shoulder to shoulder in
> the presence of an army in mutiny, can subdue the last dire enemy
> and deliver the populations not only from Asiatic cholera but from
> the immemorial fevers of the East.
>
> —William Farr, *Report on the*
> *Cholera Epidemic of 1866 in England*

WE HAVE SEEN THAT the mapping of disease operated as part of an extensive
spatialization of social knowledge which, in turn, was part of a reconceptualization of the space of the nation, the city, and the metropole. Dickens works
hard to break down the geographic conception of otherness within England
in favor of a potentially equally homogenous, equally civilized and malleable
modern urban space. But this reconceptualization of social space extended
beyond the boundaries of London or even the island. Just as St. James's was
understood in relation to its "twin," the metropole defined and was defined by
empire, and as London's space was increasingly defined in terms of its potential utopian homogeneity and abstraction, India was increasingly seen as London's double—intractably barbaric, a space defined by a fallen and changeless
geography. Epidemic disease, and especially cholera, was, by its nature,
defined as an invader, and of course cholera, coming from Bengal, was particularly subject to British scrutiny in India itself.

One might expect a similar mapping of cholera in India to that seen in
Britain; in fact, however, sanitary and cholera mapping in India follow a rather

different trajectory, one that is in dialogue with that of insular Britain, but does not parallel it directly. In part, this reflected local political investments and, of course, the limitations of a different scale. But this different history also embodies a differential understanding of space between metropole and colony, a different way of both perceiving and conceiving that space and thus of representing it. It is appropriate here to make a detour in the narrative of metropolitan mapping which we have traced, to examine the impact of British medical and sanitary spatial representation in the colony which was so important to the story of nineteenth-century cholera; and it is appropriate as well that this story fits only obliquely with the story of spatial representation at the metropole. For British India was both a separate entity, with its own political, administrative, and representational challenges, and a relative creature, defined persistently against an England which was the ideal of home to its administrators and which was the actual base of administrative power. In turn, however, India became an imagined space having some power to define the metropole as well.

This chapter will provide an overview of cholera in British India and British attitudes toward it. It will also include a survey of the fairly promising beginnings of cholera mapping in India, which were consonant with such mappings elsewhere in the world. British medics in India initially saw an opportunity to contribute to European knowledge about this important disease, and also to claim professional standing based on their intimate experience of the disease. In this, they were much like their insular counterparts. However, insular resistance to these voices caused these medics to fail in their ambition in the short term. Ironically, by the time insular medics were listening, medical mapping in India had diverged considerably from its early roots.

CHOLERA IN BRITISH INDIA

Although medics had traced the geographical progress of cholera from India even in the first epidemic of 1832, there was at that time very little attempt to fix geographical blame for the epidemic. In part because disease was not thought by medics to be caused by a specific entity, contagionism was much more powerful at the common sense level of discourse than among British medics until at least the mid-1850s. Early on, although some did argue that cholera was the disease endemic to India and traceable in its progress from east to west, there was a good deal of debate about whether "Asiatic" cholera wasn't really just a virulent strain of "English cholera" or autumnal diarrhoea. Even by the third epidemic (which struck Britain in 1854–55), when it was generally understood to have originated in India, emphasis was on the European version; a widely quoted *Lancet* article suggested that the modifier "Asiatic" should be dropped, since the disease was so strongly entrenched in England and should be studied in its manifestations specific to that area. To the extent that the disease spread in London, the "filthy" parishes of the East and South were largely to be held responsible (and by implication, their often Irish or other foreign residents).

However, by 1866, the disease is referred to almost exclusively as "Asiatic" or "Indian" cholera; the conclusion of the International Sanitary Conference was that "the whole odium of being cholera producers has been thrown on our Indian possessions" (Abot, 1). At the same time, descriptions of the "filthy" parishes had come to situate them in an imaginary other to England—a "heathen" country submerged under and concealed within the otherwise healthy English metropolitan heart of Empire. Control of the social body, through sanitary science and other biopolitical *savoirs*, to use Foucault's term, had by this time become both a goal of liberal government and the measure of its success. Containment of disease is equated with civilization and Englishness, pitted against a threat of racial degeneration and social anarchy. It is important to understand the degree to which British national identity depended on India as an other against and through which to define itself. As Anne McClintock puts it,

> Imperialism is not something that happened elsewhere—a disagreeable fact of history external to Western Identity. Rather, imperialism and the invention of race were fundamental aspects of Western, industrial modernity. The invention of race in the urban metropoles . . . became central not only to the self-definition of the middle class but also to the policing of the "dangerous classes." (5)

Race and geography were closely tied, and though race had been significant to epidemiological writings in the United States since at least the yellow fever epidemics of the nineteenth century's early years, there had been little crossover into British writings on epidemic disease within Britain. After the midcentury, that changes. Perhaps as an expression of Britain's ambivalent relationship to its imperial holdings, cholera comes to be seen as an invader from India. Fuelled in part by fears that the disease might become endemic to England if it had a chance to settle in the subsoil—in other words, that it might colonize British land—British authorities focused on the desirability of controlling cholera at its site of origin, a move which meant controlling the behaviors of Indians, which were supposed to produce it.

The International Sanitary Conference of 1866, which was to have a signal effect on British policy in India over the next decades, concluded that the causes of cholera were both geographical and social—geographical defects aggravated by human behavior. The conference gave the following possible reasons for its origin in India:

The principal . . . [hypothesis] consists in attributing the endemicity of cholera in Bengal to the alluvium of the Ganges and the Brahmapootra,— an alluvium rendered more particularly deleterious, under a scorching climate, by the fermentation of animal and vegetable detritus. . . . It is added, that the custom of the Hindoos of abandoning to the current of the sacred river their half-burnt corpses may explain the privilege of endemicity which the Delta of the Ganges possesses. (Abot 15)

Finally, however, the conference determines that it is human activity which starts epidemics, resulting in the following resolution: *"pilgrimages are, in India, the most powerful of all the causes which concur in the development and the propagation of epidemics of cholera"* (Abot 23, emphasis in original). Against medical theories predominating in Britain in the first three epidemics, the conference was contagionist, concluding that the epidemic is carried by man, which casts management of disease as a management of dangerous bodies and their movements. John Macpherson, in a tract entitled *Cholera in its Home*, remarks of India, "The idea has been broached that we should endeavor to stamp out cholera in its birthplace—that if we are to strike at the root of the disease, we must attack it in its home" (138), but, he adds, this is impossible because of the nature and scope of the problem; cholera is inextricable from the colonial landscape.[1]

Ramasubban observes that, in response to the Mutiny or Rebellion of 1857, vast numbers of British soldiers were sent to India (39). High death rates for these new soldiers led to some sanitary improvement for the remainder. David Arnold notes that one-third of British troop casualties after 1857 were from cholera ("Cholera and Colonialism" 127). However, Indian communities were neglected by British sanitary reformers. Vijay Prashad argues that the dominant European model of the modern state as the social body, already difficult in Europe to coordinate with classed and gendered individual bodies, conflicted in India with the "Manichaean" racial/colonial divide: black bodies could not be mapped onto a European social body. A segregated society developed of relatively hygienic British communities set at a distance from native towns left to suffer unimproved sanitation. But, as Ramasubban notes, although Britain had made its first organized enquiries into Indian sanitary conditions in 1861 (43), sweeping and expensive changes were "beyond the brief of a colonial government. It took the international embarrassment of Britain's being held responsible for the cholera pandemics by the International Cholera Conference of 1866 to push the government to act" (46).

Even then the British government did comparatively little, according to Ramasubban, preferring to implement segregation (50–51). Ramasubban asserts that there was a growing public demand among Indians for sanitary control. Until the late 1860s the government largely threw up its hands at the overwhelming task and allocated relatively few resources for it. According to

Mark Harrison, most sanitary education in India was the result of private philanthropic work, and much of that did garner the approval and support of some Indian elites (87–88). Although the government did take an interest in sanitation after 1860, earlier attempts to ameliorate the sanitary situation were modest, usually only at the local level, and faced complex obstacles.

Klein points out that epidemic cholera mortality in India (and worldwide) was at least partially a result of imperialism, even though the disease was endemic to India ("Imperialism" 492–94). Klein argues that the combination of new economic conditions with the mobility they sponsored and, paradoxically, the extensive water transport systems the British constructed were responsible for much of the appalling rise in Indian death rates in the mid and late nineteenth century. For example, Klein refers to a "recorded toll of 22 million between 1887 and 1954" ("Imperialism" 492), whereas Arnold estimates at least 23 million from 1865 to 1947 ("Cholera and Colonialism" 120). Modern transport systems also facilitated the spread of disease (Klein, "Death" 640; see also Klein, "Cholera, Dysentery and Development") and encouraged population movement, as did economic changes associated with modernization that depressed existing local economies ("Death" 645). Cholera in the Punjab, for example, was a relatively infrequent threat until midcentury railroad expansion there escalated its depredations (Klein, "Imperialism" 506). The canals built to modernize India were often without drainage systems ("Death" 649–50); they changed ecosystems and caused contamination of drinking water sources.[2] These ecological and economic changes also sometimes contributed to famine, which could triple the death rates of cholera epidemics (Arnold, "Social Crisis"). Indian reaction to the epidemics, although rooted in traditions of the disease that predated the British presence, still, as Arnold points out, often interpreted these new disasters in terms of imperial invasion. In one instance, for example, British soldiers were believed to have caused cholera by polluting a holy well—and it was, in fact, the soldiers who contaminated it with cholera vibrios (Arnold, "Cholera and Colonialism" 128).

Whereas low-lying, damp areas in England were seen as unhealthy and vulnerable to colonization by disease, all of India, and the people and behaviors that were mapped onto the land, were considered by many to constitute an ecological entity productive of evil. William Sanderson writes in 1866, "Cholera is known to have originated in India, which has long been well-populated, even in the prehistoric period. [. . .] Cholera could *originate* only in dense masses of population depositing excreta and other animalized matter over surfaces, from which it is carried by the percolation of the rainfall to the sources of the water supply" (10, emphasis in original). It is quite reasonable that, in a tradition extending back to Hippocrates's *De Aere,* landscape would be considered as a potential disease factor. However, for the British the actual geography of India was less important than its geography as represented in the

British imaginary. As Arnold demonstrates, "[B]y the late nineteenth century, India's incorporation into the tropics was becoming increasingly evident. Its diseases, . . . agriculture, even its people, were steadily brought within the framework of tropicality" (*Problem* 171). Mark Harrison points out that this vision of India was far from being universally accepted (*Climates and Constitutions* 69). And, of course, this totalizing view was much less prevalent in India itself, wherein British locals made clear distinctions between the "salubrious" hill areas and the steaming lowlands. Yet, as the century progressed, early metropolitan admiration of India's lush and varied beauty gave way to a more jaundiced and less nuanced view. At the same time, in the metropole, as Alan Bewell notes, slums and factories were being similarly tropicalized: hot, steamy, and crowded, they artificially produced the miasmatic environment that was figured as natural in the tropics (274–75). Bewell argues, using Dickens's description of Coketown as an example, that the tropics, and often colonial India, "provides the appropriate analogue for this new kind of urban space" (273). British poverty was read as replicating bad colonial geography, just as by the mid- to late century, the bodies of the British poor would be themselves racialized as other. The fact that this othering was considered artificial in Britain, however, meant that it was seen as meliorable. That this racial and geographical otherness was considered natural to the periphery meant to many that it was unchangeable.

Economically and agriculturally then, India was being assimilated into a geographical model that suited the metropole. Ironically, British deforestation and irrigation literally made parts of the environment more tropical in the negative sense the term had acquired for Europeans, which then justified domination of Indians, who were believed to be the racially degenerate products of such an environment. In 1852 William Farr wrote,

> [T]he history of the nations on the Mediterranean, on the plains of the Euphrates and Tigris, the deltas of the Indus and the Ganges, and the rivers of China, exhibits this great fact—the gradual descent of races from the high lands, their establishment on the coasts in cities sustained and refreshed for a season by immigration from the interior; their degradation in successive generations under the influence of the unhealthy earth, and their final ruin, effacement, or subjugation by new races of conquerors. The causes that destroy individual men, lay cities waste which in their nature are immortal, and silently undermine eternal empires. ("Influence of Elevation" 174)

Farr thus provides a neat justification for imperialism, as well as staking Britain's racial claims to leadership on its public health and its geography.

Farr explains that the cholera is the warning, sent by God (or Natural Law, His instrument), that the British community is also in danger of this elevation-related degeneration because so many have settled near the Thames:

"[T]he pestilence speaks to nations, in order that greater calamities than the death of the population may be averted. For to a nation of good and noble men Death is a less evil than the Degradation of Race" ("Influence of Elevation" 178). Britain, however, Farr explains, produces most of its population from high and salubrious areas; as for the rest, it could be fixed: "With wealth, industry and science at command, it is still possible to drain, and supply with pure water and a purer air, districts such as Southwark, Westminster, Liverpool and Hull" (*Report on the Mortality* xcviii).[3] This vision of an improvable Britain was based on the idea that British geography was in pretty good shape as it was, being basically good raw material with a few flaws. This improvement was not just a matter of correcting these defects, however, but of allowing human development toward perfection: "[L]et these human sacrifices suffice. The great Sanatory Reforms which will shield the country from pestilence, while they save the lives of thousands, will prevent the degradation of successive generations; and promote the amelioraton and perfection of the human race" (*Report on the Mortality* xcviii).

For Farr, race was not biologically essential in the sense that we understand that term today, being produced by the environment, but some environments were better than others, and therefore some races more subject to this teleology of perfection than others:

> The existence of the present living races has been rendered possible by processes and formations in the earliest geological eras; and the remotest generations of men are indissolubly connected in our immortal race, susceptible of an indefinite, glorious development. . . . Organic matter must be carried to the raised ground and high lands by man. There he must dwell. In fulfilling this law, he escapes from the terrible pestilence, retains his health, exalts his race, and has the fairest opportunity of recovering that Divine Image after which he is continually aspiring. (*Report on the Mortality* xcviii)

That race was geologically produced refers primarily to drainage, elevation, and dryness. Although this vision liberally embraces a universal family of humanity, there is some implication that this family has diverged considerably, based on the geology of its geography, and so some peoples have more catching up to do than others, if they are not, in fact, a lost cause.

As Arnold points out, although India never became a "neo-Europe" in Crosby's sense, the European impact on the land and people was nonetheless profound (*Problem* 176). If, as Arnold notes, these environmental representations became "a powerful emotional rallying point and a focus for an emerging sense of national identity" for India (*Problem* 185), they were equally important for British nationalism. In practically every text in which a Briton denounces Indian environment is included an explicit favorable comparison with northern Europe in general, and often Britain in particular. Indian tropicality was necessary for

Britain's sense of its superiority and right to rule. Bengal came to represent the Indian landscape for many Britons, and Bengal, a low-lying, moist, warm delta, was envisioned by the midcentury as the very type of diseased geography, insusceptible of remediation.

This sense of the difference of the two geographies kept the progress of medical knowledge in the two locations quite separate, at least initially. One might think that British medics at home, facing a new disease, would have placed a premium on the advice of medics experienced with the cholera in India. In fact, there was relatively little crossover between their work until the midcentury, when the massive influx of troops after the rebellion and the expansion of the profession made what would be called "tropical medicine" an emerging field. Although many medics working in India published in Britain during the early 1830s, in letters to *The Lancet* and the like, many if not most British medics in Britain dismissed their advice, suggesting that cholera on European terrain and in a European population in that terrain was a very different disease process than it was in India.

This attitude was consonant with beliefs about disease at the time, but it was also likely influenced by an attitude among domestic medics ranging from patronizing to contemptuous of their colleagues in India. As Harrison notes, most medics in the Indian Service were lower middle class, lower than most British civilians in India in the first half of the century, who tended to be professionals. Also, medics "considered employment in one of the uniformed medical services as a last resort, comparable with . . . the Poor Law medical service in Britain" (Harrison 31). Although tropical medicine became more central to medical knowledge in the mid-century, and of more interest regarding cholera as medics came closer to theories that accepted a specific disease agent, thus garnering a measure of respect at home for these medics' expertise, progress in the two regions' knowledge did not always coincide. Practitioners in India were more strongly and earlier inclined to contagionism than in the metropole, and when they stood on their experience, could be perceived as arrogant. When Cuningham, a practitioner from India, spoke to the Royal Medical and Chirurgical Society in London in 1874, a correspondent to the *British Medical Journal* complained that he "had been 'arrogant' and 'dismissive of all cholera research in Britain over the last 100 years'" (in Harrison 110).

Even though cholera's endemicity to India confirmed many insular prejudices about the Indian landscape and people, the conference's findings were overall unwelcome to Britons, since they involved British responsibility for containing this product of their possessions. Farr's 1868 *Report* gives an overall history of the disease and of theories. Of the origin of cholera, he has this to say:

> Like species of the animal kingdom plagues lie hidden in the strata of past history; they live, they flourish, they perish like organic forms, because they

are in their essence successive generations of organic forms at enmity with the corpuscles of which the human race consists. If the algid cholera can be spontaneously generated in Asia, why . . . not . . . in Africa, in Europe, in America? We know the summer cholera is generated in London [say the anti-contagionists]. . . . Why resort to the theory of importation? . . . [But] it is difficult looking at the chain of evidence to refuse the conviction that cholera came from Asia. (lxxxi)

Farr refers to the International Sanitary Conference, agreeing with most of their findings but arguing that quarantine is out of the question in large cities. Quarantine, of course, with its attendant expenses and difficulties, its interference with trade, was one reason the theory of contagion had been rejected early on in Britain—initial quarantines were dropped, probably in response to mercantile pressures. (Farr also refers to the conference's charge that the British government was negligent in tending its hydraulic works, but he claims this charge was dropped early on.) The conference attempted to impose quarantine regulations in the Red Sea, cutting Egypt off from all except mail contact with the West during epidemic prevalence.[4] Although Farr insists England is not on trial before Europe, the conference clearly decided that England was responsible for India and its cholera. But the task of sanitary remediation, Farr insists, though enormous, can be achieved with the cooperation of its native population:

> The men who won an empire, and stood shoulder to shoulder in the presence of an army in mutiny, can subdue the last dire enemy and deliver the populations not only from Asiatic cholera but from the immemorial fevers of the East. . . . [Drainage and irrigation must go forward.] At the risk of offending the susceptibilities which sustain [Indians'] stupendous theology, the fatal error of throwing their dead bodies . . . into the rivers from which their waters are drawn must be abandoned; other practices must be changed . . . ; and the cities, the pilgrimage, the religious festivals must be brought under regulation . . . to secure the nations of the world from evils against which they have a right to demand protection. . . . To render the generation of great epidemics of cholera rare, nay impossible, India has only to carry out the measures which have proved efficacious in England. (Farr, *Report on the Cholera* lxxxix–xc)

But this task was to prove more daunting than Farr envisioned. A number of sanitary schemes were enacted, some quite successfully, at the local level. And as Bewell also remarks, Britons sense of India as a diseased landscape implied also a colonial remediation in the earlier part of the century, when it was seen as quite analogous to British urban slums. Britain would bring the Indian landscape into the nineteenth century (Bewell 42). However, later in the century, this optimism about the tractability of the Indian landscape fades as India and Indians come to be seen as radically other. As Mark Harrison observes, "guarded optimism about acclimatization and the colonization of India prior to 1800, gave way to pessimism and the alienation of Europeans from the Indian environment; a shift which was closely related to the emergence of ideas of race and the consolidation of colonial rule" (*Climates* 3).

Since, by the 1860s, the world's attention was very much focused on India as the seat of cholera, it is useful to see how British medics in India mapped the disease previous to and during this period and how those maps were used and influenced in turn by insular readers. Two kinds of maps are favored by writers on cholera in India in the period from 1817 through roughly the midcentury: date-spot maps and maps showing lines of spread. The first is a map of all or part of India, with dates of the commencement of disease marked on locations. The second type has lines of spread marked on it, often with arrows to show direction. Sometimes this type also includes dates written next to place names. The lines are shown as either following the roads or simply as straight lines connecting places. World maps, or maps of Asia and Europe, tend to fall into the same two categories as the India maps. Often both kinds are used to suggest contagion, and this is especially true of maps with lines of spread. (Spot maps, without dates, especially those with a one-to-one ratio of symbol to death, tend to be used for sanitarian arguments, and so they are accordingly popular in England. They are also typically used with smaller areas.) In India one rarely sees such maps used; instead maps with dates or with lines connecting cases are used, and it is rare to find attempts to quantify numbers of deaths using spots.

Several accounts of the cholera in India focussing on the 1817–19 epidemic are written by British medical practitioners in India, who then recognize a potential audience in Britain in the years of spread of the 1830s epidemic. Toward the end of the first decade of the nineteenth century, many British medics in India compiled a good deal of data which was largely ignored by their counterparts at home when the 1817 epidemic never materialized in the United Kingdom. A flurry of hopeful republication of this material in Britain around the 1832 epidemic died down not long after 1833. Often these medics, such as Christie, worked for the East India Company; others, such as Orton, were affiliated with the army. Many times these works refer in their prefaces to British lack of interest in the disease before the 1830s and, more obliquely, to the scorn of British practitioners in the Isles for practitioners in India. Indeed, they were subsequently to find that even in the 1830s, insular medics tended to rely more on their own experience with European diseases they confidently expected would be similar to the new menace than on the experience of their brethren overseas.

Still, although this was a widespread attitude among insular medics, it was by no means universal, and as cholera steadily resisted treatment, insular medics became more interested in the Indian experience, especially by the midcentury. Farr and Snow, among others, took a very active interest in the Indian documents, as did many medics who worked most insightfully with maps. Others resisted one or both of these trends. By the 1860s, however, with the rise in the number of British medics going to India and the international attention given to India as the epicenter of disease, the dismissive attitude toward the work of British medics in India was on the wane, although it still varied widely according to beliefs about etiology, and so forth. Because they placed India at the center of their maps, and also included smaller maps of towns or encampments, British medics in India from 1817 to the early 1830s represented India in a very different way than did insular medics, who tended to include India, if they did at all, simply as the source of epidemics and as the far eastern point of the world of which Europe was first the western bound- ary, and sometimes later, the center, as the Americas came to take up the left limit of the map. Anglo-Indian mapping concerns continued to be quite dif- ferent, since later maps formally and visually attended to the differences between native and European mortality which had only been covered in the verbal narrative before, as British policy moved increasingly toward separating native and European sanitary concerns. The political history of British sani- tary improvement in India can be read in these reports and maps, and the rep- resentation of Indian geography in these maps, especially when compared to trends in British insular mapping, reflected and perhaps shaped the attitudes of Britons toward India and colonial disease.

INDIAN MAPS

British disease maps in the early part of the period are mostly produced with- out reference to preexisting maps. Early on in the nineteenth century, the gen- eral attitude of the British was far more accepting and respectful of Indian forms of knowledge than by midcentury. Bewell observes that, as opposed to the racialized views of the later nineteenth century, the early period is marked by a sense of the parity of the British urban poor and the colonial sufferer (270). Many British medics sought out and tried native remedies, and often they found their way into permanent use. Why didn't British medics use native maps? Surprisingly, in the recent spate of scholarship dealing with the mapping of India, there is little attention to the relationship between indige- nous mapping and European mapping of India. Edney's excellent book gives little on the prehistory of European mapping, pointing put merely that Britons distrusted and dismissed Indian conceptions of space and had little faith in their ability to adopt Western standards of accuracy. He notes that early European maps of India relied a good deal on Indian information, but always discarded it as soon as information collected by Europeans was available, even if the native material was accurate by Western standards (309).[5] In fact, there was indeed an indigenous tradition of mapping and geographic discourse, which influenced and, at least at some postmedieval point, was unevenly influenced by Chinese, Middle Eastern, North African, and European mapping. But the purpose of such mapping differed from the purpose of British mapping by the late eighteenth century, when most imperial mapping was done, and so the native traditions passed out of the sphere of what was constructed as active geographical knowledge and into that of antiquarianism and ethnohistory. By the time medical maps were made, the mapping tradition in India, or what was identified as such, was fully Westernized. Still, the written tradition of geographic knowledge continued to be influential until quite late, not being eliminated completely until the entire country was mapped using new methods of triangulation.[6]

The denial of the native tradition, and the dismissal of the detailed geographical history that was inseparable from geography in the Puranas, reconstructed India as a land without a history or a historiography, a mute or a nonexistent cartographic tradition. It is this view which is reflected in the British maps we see for at least the first six decades of the nineteenth century. Despite written evidence that rivers had changed course over the years and so on, none of these changes seem to be tracked in the British disease maps of India in the first half of the nineteenth century, which fixed the land as a de novo object found by British mappers. Perhaps partially for this reason, we see no attempts to layer the maps, as in Oxford or St. James's (although this is probably also an issue of scale), to compare the courses of illness and the changes that have taken place over time, sanitary or otherwise. As in the texts we have examined, India is presented as a land either without history or a land with too much history—either way, it seems that the layering of the history of the land is not a narrative of progress or change, but a static narrative of repetition, the crushing weight of sameness infinitely repeated, following some decay which is vaguely assumed to have taken place before European arrival. In fact, many British medics in the first half of the century did write medical topographies, especially of areas important to the East India Company, and some of these could have been resourced to provide a more layered history and mapping of India, but none seem to have been used for this, despite their fairly widespread availability (Farr mentions having read most of these treatises in the mid-1850s).[7] But most of the readers of these studies seem to have been insular ones.

It is true that medical topographies were selectively produced for a few areas with large European populations; however, they were at least available and continued to be published until the mid-1850s, whereupon production seems to have largely ceased. Mark Harrison makes the useful point that there is a dual tradition in such representations: local maps and medical topographies may be quite detailed and represent the land as quite salubrious, especially in the highlands, whereas larger scale representations move in the opposite direction (e-mail correspondence, Dec. 2002). However, none of the official reports even of the 1860s or cholera maps seem to have consulted these works, and there seems generally to be little interest in showing an historical progression. There are a number of possible reasons for this—most cholera maps are constructed by medical officers, not by historians or cartographers, for example. It is not my intention to argue that these mapmakers consciously set out to display India as a land without history, although it seems clear that for these mappers, Indian history was at least irrelevant to any notion of Western history as a record of progression toward modernity. However, regardless of intention, that is the effect these maps promote. They are clearly not designed to initiate the kinds of large sanitary reform projects their insular counterparts were. In other words, we don't see an implicit conceived space of order and transparency to which the perceived space is compared and toward which a developmental narrative can be envisioned. As we shall see, this trend both culminated and was challenged in the years immediately following the International Sanitary Conference, when mappers were highly motivated either to imagine the possibility of sanitary change for the first time, or to resist it; in turn, Indian maps, for the first time, began to reflect the possibility of a geographical narrative not merely based on iteration, but on historical change.

EARLY MAPS BY BRITISH MEDICS IN INDIA

Early British medical mappers in India were, by and large, genuinely interested in the disease and its geography; their maps were state of the art and differ little from those created in Europe.[8] Both European and overseas mappers worked largely in world maps. Domestic maps tended to be for the whole country, so were fairly large scale. Only city maps were lacking from the British Indian archive, largely because the mappers concerned were tracing data for entire residencies. This is also a period in which much less hostility and contempt for native traditions informs British writing than in later years; Indians (at least in the higher castes) are still represented as cleanly, and native remedies are considered with some respect as potentially efficacious, if unscientific. Principally, then, medics in these texts attempt to describe the disease, rather than a diseased landscape or inherently diseased population. They also, like medics at home, use their experience and expertise to position themselves as public commentators on the health of the state. In their case, however, this is usually less an attempt to communicate with the general public than to take a place in a specifically metropolitan professional landscape.

Orton is a good example of a practitioner in India who had hopes of making his mark in Britain during the 1830s epidemic. In his 1831 preface, Orton states that first edition of his book was published earlier "in a very unprepossessing form" in Madras (i), and that he had originally planned to publish another volume on the contagiousness of cholera, but "found the subject possessing but a very subdued and secondary degree of interest" in England" (xiv). Obviously he believes that insular medics will find his work more interesting as cholera marches across the European continent toward Britain. The map shows most of the Indian subcontinent and places with dates of first appearance of cholera;[9] it bears the legend "Map exhibiting the progress of The Epidemic Cholera over the principal parts of India, by the dates of its first appearance at numerous places with the great roads &c." The result of this scheme of representation is that Orton shows places hit by cholera only, and shows them connected only by roads. He shows no other roads (that is, between places not affected by the disease). Not all dates show the year, although it appears that where the year is not shown, it is 1818. May 15 is the earliest date shown, in Vizagapatam. Although the entire map does not show clear a progression in dates along the roads, several areas clearly do (for example from Calcutta down the coast to Trichinopoly, fig. 6.1).

The map is thus heavily weighted towards contagionism and by using the roads to show connections between stricken areas, implies that the cholera spread thereby. Orton states:

> The doctrine of contagion in general has gained very little support in India [regarding most diseases]. . . . It was therefore not without astonishment that many of the profession in India heard that the Medical Board of Bombay, in 1818, held the disease to be contagious. My feeble voice, in common with the great majority, was raised in opposition to the—as it appeared—monstrous dogma; but the march of time and events, the great accumulation of facts and gradual removal of prejudices, have wrought in my mind the same revolution that they have in so many others. The opinion of the contagious nature of the disease has been gradually gaining ground even in India, and seems to be the general one in Europe. Veritas magna est et praevalebit. (314)

Of course, this British Indian "consensus," if ever there was one, (and Christie claims just the opposite, mentioning that belief in noncontagion was almost universal) was out of favor in Britain, which may account in part for Orton's lack of popularity there. Truth took an inordinately long time to prevail, its greatness notwithstanding. In India, however, although contagionism waxed and waned, there seemed to be a much more long lasting and prevalent sense that cholera was or might be contagious, at least contingently. Orton accounts for the epidemic's seemingly multiple points of origin by endemicity

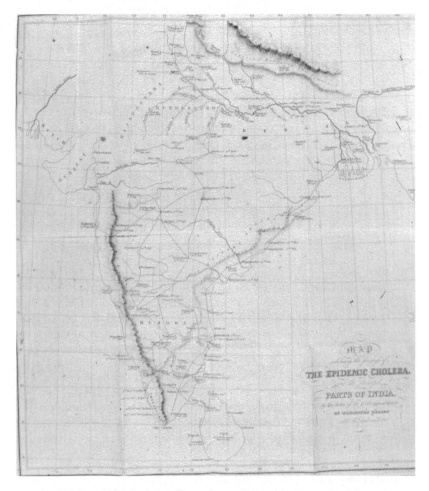

FIGURE 6.1. Orton's Map: detail. From Orton, Reginald. *An Essay on the Epidemic Cholera of India.* 2nd ed., with a supplement. Burgess and Hill: London, 1831.

and shows that it follows troop movements—another reason his work may have been received less than enthusiastically at home—in a narrative mapping of its progress which never explicitly refers to his cartogram, but may be followed there.[10]

As noted above, many India maps and world or region maps in this period are oriented toward contagion; indeed, belief in contagion was much more widespread among British practitioners in India than at home, both in the 1830s and subsequently. Still, it was never by any means universal, and may not even have enjoyed a consistent majority. Alexander Turnbull Christie, M.D., wrote *A Treatise on the Epidemic Cholera*, which was published in London in 1833. He worked for the East India Company, and was also a member of the Royal Asiatic Society of Great Britain and Ireland. Like many others, he first published his work locally in India (in 1828), and then tried for the insular market. Christie was anticontagionist, yet he uses a map much like the maps his colleagues were creating and upon which it was probably modeled— that is, one with dates on onset—and found himself immediately at odds with it, since this format tends to support a contagionist argument. He seemed to feel, however, that the inclusion of a map was de rigueur.

Christie's map was entitled "Map of the Countries visited by the Epidemic Cholera from the Year 1817 to the Year 1830, inclusive; with the dates of its first appearance at the principal places attacked by it." He almost never refers to the map, except in one notable passage in which he denounces it as a form of representation unsuited to its topic:

> Upon casting the eye over it, it may appear that the disease has generally followed the course of great rivers, or of frequented lines of communication between different countries; but this is more in appearance than reality, and is owing to various causes. 1st. In all countries the cities and large towns are situated on rivers or on great roads; and these naturally engross our attention, while the villages in the intermediate spaces are neglected [and it is impossible, even if data were available, to include them for reasons of space]. . . . [I]t would be hardly possible to represent, with perfect accuracy and in detail, its exact progress through the country, its quick passage . . . and its sudden appearance and disappearance; but it may be figured to the imagination as a winged restless fiend, hovering over a country and alighting occasionally, and in a capricious mood, to contaminate with his hateful presence the air immediately around. Not to make the map an inconvenient size, it has been necessary to make the equator its Southern limit [so infected places South are not represented]. (3–4)

One sees here the frustration of a not particularly cartographically savvy person who has tried constructing a map, using what he thought of as standard techniques without any sense of their argumentative investments, and has found the "objective" representation contradicts his representational purposes. (He would have been far better off with a spot map.) In fact, Christie wrote in quite a few names of villages (with dates of cholera onset) which were not on the original map, so his argument that small settlements are left out appears to be the voice of experience. However, his map does not appear to be comprehensive in its coverage of these villages either, and it is not clear whether he simply gave up writing them in after attempting it, or whether the ones he has chosen to include were selected according to some unstated principle.

Significantly, Christie's narrative of the cholera's spread—filled with words like "capricious," "sudden," and the like, in contradiction to other writers' (e.g., Scot's) narratives of inexorable if uneven spread—exhorts the reader to forget the map, to fill the mind's eye instead with the imaginative representation of a "winged fiend," evoking instead of the map the many imaginative iconic representations of cholera in European newspapers as a winged and cloaked skeleton flying over stricken communities. Christie distrusts not only the map's selectivity but also its tendency to actively participate in the construction of a contagionist argument, as other maps have apparently tended to do. The man on the ground, he asserts, has intimate knowledge as valuable as the abstract overview generated from the bird's-eye perspective, or perhaps more. This amounts to a denial of the basis of legitimation for mapping—its objective viewpoint, its clinical detachment—in fact, a denial of abstraction as a principle for both understanding and change. However, this is an isolated argument against maps by one who has clearly thought deeply about their limits, learned in the process of constructing one.

The two most important cholera maps of this period in terms of their later influence are those by Scot and Jameson. Surgeon William Scot's 1824 *Report on the Epidemic Cholera as it has appeared in the territories subject to The Presidency of Fort St. George* is a folio volume, and includes a map about two inches wider than the volume itself. The map is a more professional job than Christie's or Jameson's. Hand drawn and colored, with some attention to aesthetics (mountain ranges are green, the ocean is blue), it uses red and yellow lines to show the progress of the disease.[11] The text refers to the map: "The narrative and the map . . . will clearly evince, that the progress of the disease from North to South, has been affected with surprising regularity both geographically and chronologically" (xlvi). This north-south model, although it comes up sporadically, never seems to have caught on; by the midcentury it was a rarely challenged truism that not only cholera, but epidemics generally, moved from east to west. Scot does not seem to have republished an insular version for the 1832 epidemic, waiting instead until the third epidemic in 1849 to publish an abridged report with Blackwood, in Edinburgh. Here, he notes that the "greater part of the first edition [of 1824] was reserved for India, and only a limited number of copies transmitted to the India house for distribution in this country. It was the last published of the official reports" (i). He explains that the many tables, sick returns, and so on

> unfortunately swelled the Madras report to the inconvenient size of a folio volume of 550 pages, rendering it altogether inaccessible to the medical profession in Britain [and only known through reviews which appeared at the time of publication]. . . . When cholera afterwards found its way to Europe, and afforded to every man the means of forming his own opinion . . . hopes

were entertained that the researches of so great a body of able and scientific men as Britain possessed, would lead to a more perfect knowledge of a disease which had too much baffled the efforts of their brethren in India. (ii)

But that, as Scot observes, didn't happen, and now, he writes, the publication of an accessible version might be a service to British medics, since it is founded on the authority of massive empirical evidence. One senses a good deal of irony in his generally tactful summing up of British practitioners' dismissal of the clinical experience of Anglo-Indian medics in favor of an overweening confidence in their own, defeated, medical knowledge. In the work of many practitioners in India publishing in Britain in the 1830s, there was a sense that this was the moment to make claims for their own specialized knowledge and the value of their skills as scientific observers. The success of this move was somewhat equivocal; it would be many years before such medics were given the same respect as their insular counterparts. Still, some did read their work, and by the midcentury, they were often cited. Scot clearly senses that this is a moment to try again, insular medics having been sufficiently chastened by their inability to conquer the disease.

Scot's 1849 "Narrative of the Progress of the epidemic cholera in the peninsula of India" runs from pages 148 to 212 in a book totalling 212 pages *(Report on the Epidemic Cholera)*. In the main body of the text Scot dutifully focuses more on meteorological data than contagion theories. However, his map, which is inscribed on a preprinted map showing the middle to southern portion of India only (the northernmost large towns shown on the map are Surat, Pandhoorna, and Sumbulpoor) with all principal roads clearly marked, shows roads marked with two colors: red, for roads where cholera had definitely spread on the road between two towns, and yellow, crossroads between two places where cholera had spread, but could not be ascertained to have been suffered by victims on the road (see fig. 6.2). Unlike Orton's map or Scot's own earlier one, which only traces the roads and towns pertaining to cholera routes, this map, inscribed onto an up-to-date survey map, shows all roads and larger towns.[12] Dates of commencement are inscribed in a larger, slightly darker script under the place-names. Because Scot's inking follows the roads, again, the overwhelming impression is one of contagion.[13]

This map is considerably more detailed than the map Scot uses in his earlier, more massive report. It is notable that although Scot condenses the text, he does not bother to update it significantly, nor include data beyond that originally available in 1824—but he updates the map, inscribing the lines and dates on the more accurate and detailed map of the late 1840s. There is, however, some carelessness in reproduction; for example, the yellow line from Hoogly to Darwar, and the date of attack in Hoogly (August 13) drop out, despite remaining references to Hoogly in the narrative (Scot 1849, 164).

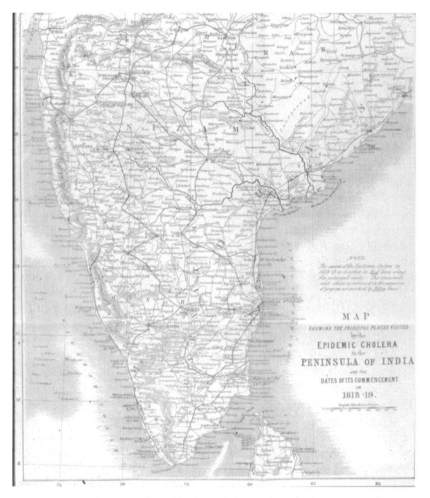

FIGURE 6.2. Scot's Map: detail. From Scot, William. *Report on the Epidemic Cholera as it has appeared in the territories subject to The Presidency of Fort St. George.* Drawn up by order of government, under the superintendence of the medical board. Abridged from the original report printed at Madras in 1824, with introductory remarks, by the author. Edinburgh: William Blackwood and Sons, 1849. Image reproduced by permission of The Wellcome Library, London.

However, he does add a thirty-one-page prefatory remarks section to the text, which responds to other writers (not, generally, by name) and rather pointedly remarks upon the tendency of insular medics to disregard the work of British medics in India. He considers it probable that "the ganglionic system of nerves form the primary seat of the disease" (ix) and notes that "the doctrine that cholera depended on 'a diminished energy of the nervous system . . .' . . . was laid down in the Madras report (page 76 of the present edition) and yet we find it claimed as a discovery in this country" and, he adds, the same has happened with the term "cholera asphyxia"(x).

He also uses the preface to remark on the tendency in Britain to claim that cholera is not contagious and refute it. He notes that cholera appears to follow watercourses, and that this has been used in sanitary arguments, as the poor tend to live close to watercourses and in filthy circumstances. However, he maintains that the conditions of poverty themselves are debilitating to health, as is dirt, but that dirt is not a cause of disease per se (xiv), a sentiment that Snow would echo a few years later after careful consideration of the work of medics in India. He also pointedly mentions the prevailing wisdom that plagues invade the clean and innocent West from the decadent East: "It has been said, that all our fatal epidemics have come from the East; but . . . the influenza came to India from the West," and elsewhere in his narrative, he shows that the cholera also moved further east from India. Here we see that British medics in India used maps not only to communicate information, but also to legitimate themselves as professionals and to challenge insular stereotypes about both Indian life and practice.

These maps were later to become important to John Snow and William Acland in their own research, so perhaps Scot got his wish at last. But as late as 1873, Acland still felt the need to assert that he looked on "Indian sanitary work as one with our own, and invaluable as affording a means of comparison amongst various races. I hope the day will come, when this is so far understood, that an interchange of duties may take place between British and Indian Sanitary Officers" (*Health* vi). Even in the 1870s, such a connection between the two professional groups was not automatic; additionally, by the 1870s the assumptions of parity in the disease and in the population had been lost. Acland values the Indian sanitary service for its ability to "compare . . . races," a project which did not occur to Scot and his contemporaries, who largely saw differences in disease as related more to climate than to the biological sense of race which is emerging at the time Acland speaks.

James Jameson's *Report on the Epidemick Cholera Morbus, as it Visited the Territories subject to the Presidency of Bengal in the Years 1817, 1818, and 1819*, published in 1820, has a relatively uninteresting map, simply showing place names of where cholera prevailed and rivers in a small section of India for which he is responsible. The land exceeds the margins of the map, and Jameson has little interest in the depredations of the epidemic beyond his own bailiwick. Not including dates, it operates more like a spot map, in accord with his sanitary argument. Jameson's report is unique in this period in that it takes a sanitary point of view very early, in opposition to any con-

tagionist position, and implicates Indian native practices with marked dis-
taste (though he does also see wind as a significant factor): "[A] great mischief consequent on the intermixture of European and Native dwellings
[caused by the rise of population sparked by the consolidation of the Empire
in Calcutta], has been the accumulation of filth in every vacant space"
(110–11). He then gives a sanitary narrative of the center of the city and
calls for sanitary reforms, including increased drainage, sewerage, and so
forth. He mentions the Hurdwar pilgrimage as having been a focal point of
the disease some years earlier, though he blames it on sleeping in the cold
rather than on filth (xvi–xvii). He sees natives and Europeans as constitutionally different, which is again rare in documents from this place and
period, considering most natives as having less hardy constitutions than
Europeans (53). He also has little use for native remedies, calling them "friv-
olous" or "pernicious" (243). Ironically, one of the methods he cites is a form
of oral rehydration therapy, using salt water, rose water, and lemonade—
exactly what would now be prescribed. He also is the only writer from India
I have found in this period who insists that the disease moves from east to
west in a very unusual way:

> From the remote period of its first appearance in the Eastern Parts of Ben-
> gal . . . to the hour of its arriving on the Malabar Coast . . . its path was
> almost uniformly from East to West. . . . It seemed so bent upon pursuing
> the Westerly course, that rather than deviate from it in an opposite direction,
> it would for a while desert a tract of country, to which it afterward returned
> under circumstances more congenial to its disposition. (96)

Given that Jameson claims it is impossible to know how cholera began or
how it is transmitted (though he is solidly anticontagionist), this is a particularly odd assertion. How would one know that the cholera had stopped
spreading "until circumstances more congenial to its disposition" were found,
and what were such circumstances? His contention that it did not go east contradicts all the evidence available about that epidemic, which spread to China,
Burma and points south. The insistence on an east to west route is significant,
as it became the dominant view of insular medics that cholera (and indeed,
that most plagues) moved in this way, and was later to become an important
part of the demonization of the East.

Jameson, perhaps because of these peculiarities, which anticipated later
British attitudes, is the early Indian authority most often cited in the 1860s in
India, and frequently in the midcentury by sanitarian reports in Britain as
well. Although his work is unusual in its time—the contempt for Indian practices and attention to sanitary problems particularly—it accorded very well
with the sanitary project in Britain and with racist views of the 1860s in both
Britain and Anglo-India, which may have had much to do with Jameson's

later popularity in comparison to, say, William Scot's work, although it was quite detailed and thorough as well, which certainly also recommended it to some medics' attention.[14]

In short, the maps of this period have some principal similarities and differences from their insular counterparts. Like them, they usually begin with a de novo mapping of the territory in question, not relating the cholera directly to other indicators (for example, poverty, fever, and so on), and like them, they tend to take a stand on the spread of cholera which is either vaguely miasmatic/weather related or contagionist, though they are far more likely to be contagionist than their insular counterparts. Like them, too, medics attempt to use them to claim or consolidate authority in the English public sphere; however, for many years, that claim would go unregarded. Finally it was Farr and Snow who, using both Scot and Jameson, would be increasingly convinced of the waterborne theory. At last, some insular medics valued the input of their colleagues abroad. However, despite the fact that these insular medics would use the Indian maps to construct a history and progression of cholera in maps which were increasingly complex and more intimately tied to diagnosis and treatment or improvement of the territory depicted, Indian maps would largely not reflect this trend until after the late 1860s. As we shall see in the next chapter, the 1860s brought conflict and change to the medical mapping of India.

7

India in the 1860s

Mapping Imperial Difference

Cholera is known to have originated in India, which has long been
well-populated, even in the prehistoric period. Cholera could *originate* only in dense masses of population depositing excreta and
other animalized matter over surfaces, from which it is carried by
the percolation of the rainfall to the sources of the water supply.

—Dr. William Sanderson, "Suggestions in Reference
to the Present Cholera Epidemic, for the Purification
of the Water Supply and the Reclamation of East London,
with Remarks on One Origin of the Cholera Poison"

THE YEARS INTERVENING BETWEEN the early 1830s and the mid-1860s produced, relatively speaking, far fewer medical maps by British medics in India
than were created at either end of the period. Mapping of India for military,
ordinance, railway building, and drainage and irrigation purposes continued
apace but, perhaps because of cholera's endemicity, and because the epidemic
years in Europe were accompanied by other upheavals (the Crimean war, for
example, and the Indian Rebellion in 1857, when some medics might still
have been collating information about the 1855 outbreak), there are relatively
few new disease maps from the midcentury included in the India Office's *Catalogue of Manuscript and Printed Reports, Field Books, Memoirs, Maps . . . of the
Indian Surveys deposited in the Map Room of The India Office* (and even fewer
are still available in Britain). There seems little doubt that, while local medical mapping expanded in the Isles, in India it flagged, perhaps in part because

of the increasing separation of native and European towns and again, because cholera's endemicity didn't give it the seemingly temporally limited character that inspired much insular mapping. Drainage maps were the closest to sanitary maps and focused on the frustratingly moist Indian terrain, often exposing cross sections of the earth under houses and showing the type of ground material. But these gave little information on disease per se. The writers of the *Report on the Cholera Epidemic of 1867 in Northern India* complain that

> Of the unusual prevalence of cholera in earlier years, no precise records are available. . . . Even of the outbreak of 1856, which in many respects resembled those of 1861 and 1867, and which was more fatal to the European troops than either of them, no general history is available. From the scanty and detached records which are to be had, it is impossible to say with any degree of accuracy which places were visited by the disease, what was the history of the epidemic, and what the losses it occasioned in each. (Malleson and Cuningham 1)

In fact, the report refers extensively to Jameson's 1817 report and little else. Townsend's 1869 report on the Central Provinces also regrets the "scanty and imperfect" data available before the 1860s. Interestingly, however, although the reports of this period tend to refer to earlier work such as Jameson's, they do not attempt to map a historical comparison as have British medics since the arrival of the second epidemic. Of course, the frequency of epidemics and uneven availability of data may have militated against this desire; still, one might think that at least locally and over the short term, medics would have been moved to produce such comparisons in the midcentury.

As mentioned earlier, the maps generated in the late 1860s show the decided impact of the International Sanitary Conference's decision that cholera is spread by human contact and has to do with native pilgrimage. The 1860s maps tend to be made with the definite purpose of investigating relatively small areas under the direct authority of the report maker, and often also attempt to exculpate the report maker from responsibility for outbreaks. Later maps tend to blame native customs, especially religious ones, and native "dirtiness" for cholera. Early mapmakers, except for Jameson, did not do this.[1] Scot mentions native customs only once, when he remarks that the excitement of a sacrifice to propitiate deities regarding cholera and overeating sacrificial meat in hot weather brought on some individuals' illness (167–68), but this is momentary, and is not emphasized as a primary cause of disease, which he believes is meteorological. Orton's interests are entirely meteorological and geological. He is more likely to blame earthquakes than human customs, although he notes that deprivation predisposes one to suffer, and that upper-class Indians suffer less than the poor (434). When he implicates human habits, it is the Russians and eastern Europeans who suffer in comparison to Britain and India:

> Let us call to mind the difference between these countries and in India. In
> the latter, the living sub dio—the free ventilation—the cleanliness—
> enforced in the case of European soldiers, and carried by the Hindoo, both
> from religion and choice, to a most scrupulous extent, form a complete con-
> trast to the habits . . . of the lower orders of Russia, Poland, & c. (462)

England, he suggests, will not suffer much, because "[o]ur lowest classes
hold a higher place, both moral and physical . . . than those of any other country, and our humane and generous poor laws render absolute want of the necessaries of life among them impossible" (474), but Ireland, he predicts, will
suffer horribly. Part of this was typical of European attitudes of the time
toward India,[2] but it is also possible that dramatic regional differences, as well
as personal differences between writers affected the perspective of the reports:
Calcutta, wherein Jameson was located, may have been far more challenging
to European tastes than Madras, as well as more medically problematic. In any
case, however, the 1860s show a marked turn to blaming.

Still, not all medics in the 1860s concentrate on or are interested in the
action of the natives. The midcentury saw a massive study of the drainage of
India and those medics most involved in ongoing drainage issues in the
1860s seem least interested in blaming anyone for outbreaks and more
focused on doing something about sanitary conditions. Of the many who do
engage in blaming Indians, it may be said that the systematic segregation of
European and native settlement following the growth of the British military
after the events of 1857 probably contributed to the othering of the native
population. The two perspectives are neatly illustrated in two very different
reports, bound together. The first is preoccupied with native activity and the
second with the land.

G. B. Malleson and J. M. Cuningham's *Report on the Cholera Epidemic of
1867 in Northern India* (1868) contains three maps. The first, "Map of Northern India to illustrate the Cholera Epidemic of 1867," is large scale—ninety-
six miles to the inch—and shows the "area covered by the epidemic," a large
portion of the upper left side of the map, with a uniform "yellow tint." A
meteorological chart is included. The text blames the epidemic on the Hurdwar Fair and attendant pilgrimage and says it did not arise out of sanitary conditions (for which the local British government was responsible). It also argues
against the sanitary position generally, asserting that cholera is not filth generated. After all, the authors observe, the natives are relatively filthy all the
time. Still, it equivocates, pleading for support for sanitation because,
although filth does not generate cholera, it is favorable to its dissemination
(138). This seems a rather clumsy way of appealing for more resources without quite admitting that lack of resources led to governmental inefficiency.
The second map is a local map of the fair showing, in color, latrines, hospitals,

boats, and a "bungalow" (see fig. 7.1). It also shows the location of police, a ghat (steps leading to the water), and a horse fair. The map follows the approved format for a sanitary map, showing potential nuisances, and so on, but the adjacent text charges the pilgrims with bringing in cholera (37).

The report finds cholera's communicability "indisputable" (131). Reinforcing this point, a line map shows the movement of pilgrims from Hurdwar Fair and the dates of first illness at each site. This line map is a rare abstract map of Indian space—it is not superimposed over a landmap, but exists solely as a connect-the-dots (see fig. 7.2). Although the map attempts correct scale, it doesn't show the shape of the land beneath it or roads, although it does show the river Indus and a section of railway connecting two stricken locations. It also indicates whether the first case in each location was, him or herself, a pilgrim (between pages 132 and 133).

In this map, the land is entirely effaced, bringing into sharp focus the spatial relationship of human actions as the only determining factor (and only native actions as disease producing). In Britain, as we have seen, abstract maps

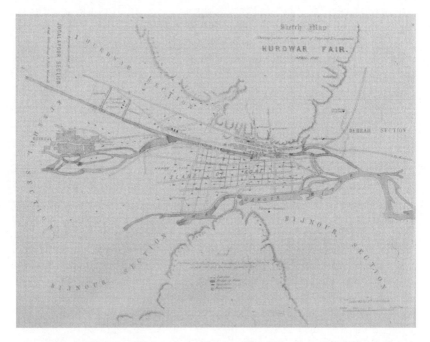

FIGURE 7.1. Malleson and Cuningham: Hurdwar Fair Map. From Malleson, G.B. and Cuningham, J.M. *Report on the Cholera Epidemic of 1867 in Northern India.* Calcutta: Office of Superintendent of Government Printing, 1868. Image reproduced by permission of The Wellcome Library, London.

operated as shorthand evoking spatial relationships which the viewer already knew (see, for example, fig. 3.8 in chapter 3). Here, however, the object is not to simplify by excluding information which will be distracting, but to obscure information which might be used for different purposes, for an audience which almost certainly did not possess the elided information, nor a detailed mental map of the area in question. The land is remapped as the neutral setting for deleterious human activities, positioned as militating against the sanitary management of the local British government. Religious activities were the favorites for scapegoating. They operated both as indices of Indian "barbarism"—Hindu pantheism, for example, as opposed to Christianity—and because the sensitivity of religious issues tended to publicly justify a laissez-faire approach to them, intervention being held likely to provoke civil unrest. (The 1857 Rebellion was widely held to have resulted from subalterns' religious objections to the use of beef and pork fat in greasing weaponry.) Coolie labor gangs, also a target of suspicion, were more problematic scapegoats since often they were following the labor market created by British industry and agriculture.

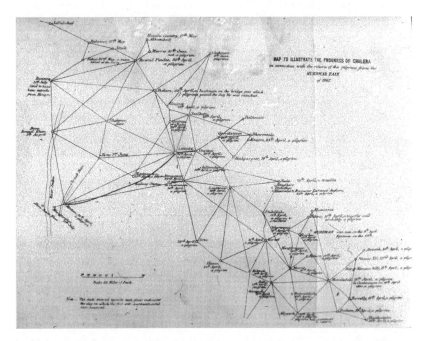

FIGURE 7.2. Malleson and Cuningham: Pilgrims Line Map. From Malleson, G.B. and Cuningham, J.M. *Report on the Cholera Epidemic of 1867 in Northern India.* Calcutta: Office of Superintendent of Government Printing, 1868. Image reproduced by permission of The Wellcome Library, London.

Malleson and Cuningham dwell at length on the customs of the natives, giving the whole history of Hurdwar Fair (believed the epicenter of the outbreak), which an estimated 3 million people attended (8), with special attention to "violence and bloodshed at former fairs" (4–5). It is clear that the fair itself is being attacked, and not solely in light of its epidemiological implications. A great deal of attention is paid to the arrangements the sanitary authorities made, and also to the cultural activities of the fairgoers, on whom, in line with the findings of the Constantinople conference, the responsibility for the outbreak will be principally placed by the authors. This writers feel that although associated with human contact, the mode of propagation is unclear (17); they focus briefly on possible contamination of the water supply by the latrines (19), but then dismiss that in favor of contamination at the ghat, where pilgrims, according to one Doctor Cutcliffe's report, drank while they bathed and gave each other water in their cupped hands as part of ritual. The natives' supposition that the illness had something to do with placing the latrines close to the sleeping quarters, where the contents might have overflowed into the soil during heavy rains, though a good example of insular British sanitary reasoning in this period, is dismissed as the reaction of an "ignorant and terrified multitude" under difficult circumstances (18). Note also that although close attention is paid to the actions of pilgrims at the fair, the larger map of the epidemic's impact effaces all subsequent human activity, showing a uniform tint rather than dates or lines of spread.

W. R. Cornish, FRCS, sanitary commissioner for Madras, published his *Report on Cholera in Southern India for the Year 1869, with map illustrative of the disease* in 1870. His report is mostly a series of charts and diagrams with a fairly brief narrative, principally concerned with English troops. That cholera is spread by pilgrims is assumed. The report is cobbled together out of various subordinates' reports, often tacked on whole as appendices, and Cornish doesn't do much with them. He refers to recently issued "more detailed instructions for investigation of cholera, drawn up by the Army Sanitary Commission and forwarded to India with the Despatch No. 10 of 23rd April 1869," which have set new standards of specificity (1). The volume includes a copy of a report by a surgeon, W. A Thompson, on cholera at Secunderabad during 1868–69. After carefully tracing all cholera cases, and adducing no evidence of communication between the European victims in married barracks and the cooly village, this surgeon is sure that it must have come from the cooly village, though how, he "can't say" (53). The map of the encampment shows no lines of communication or dots.

As is typical of the reports that rely strongly on native habits as cause of the disease, there is extensive attention to native habits, which we do not see in Balfour's report, appendixed in the same volume, for example. Interestingly, it includes a question and answer session, in an appendixed report by Thompson, with the headman of the cooly village, which provides an interesting perspective on one native's responses within a particular, and perhaps hostile, interrogatory situation. Thompson asks if the villagers think cholera is contagious, and the unnamed man answers, "The Burmese think so." The Burmese are also said to think that drinking bad water and eating bad food can cause it. Is Thompson's interlocutor using an out group with even less status as a scapegoat, or is he using them to advance an opinion which he himself holds but is not sure the British want to hear? Thompson's sole comment on the Burmese is that when cholera appeared, "[T]he Burmese fired guns, rockets and such like . . . and made all sorts of horrible noises to frighten away the demon god who was supposed to have something to do with the prevailing epidemic" (69)—a quite different vision of Burmese views on disease etiology than is revealed in the interview. In any case, the coolies, who are by now routinely charged with responsibility for the spread of cholera, provide a convenient opportunity for the British to take action. The report concludes, rather chillingly, "I am happy to state, that since writing the remarks on the condition of the cooly village in the body of the preceding report, active measures have been taken by the Civil authorities towards the removal of the said village altogether" (69).[3]

S. C. Townsend's *Report on the Cholera Epidemic of 1868* is bound with Malleson and Cuningham's report. It contains several charts and two carefully prepared maps. This report also uses yellow shading delimited in pencil to mark the cholera field in a large map of central India. Townsend takes for granted that cholera is contagious, and remarks that the local fair was cancelled because of the cholera, adding that the native population were very reasonable about the explanation. Unfortunately, Townsend remarks, travelling "cooly" labor gangs disseminated the disease anyway. However, Townsend, unlike Malleson and Cuningham, is principally interested in bad or disease producing geography, and his maps reflect that, showing little interest in human activity, despite his belief that the disease is actually spread by human agency. He shows relatively little interest in native customs, except to explain how the coolies are travelling and how various dead bodies got into various water sources; his focus is not on blaming the carriers, but considering the geological and geographical factors which favor the pollution of water and thus the spread of disease. He is interested in geographic melioration, and his report thus gives much more attention to soil composition, water sources, drainage, and the like. Townsend describes the people in the area he is responsible for with respect, if not much interest, and he is not at all motivated to blame their customs, but to improve drainage.

Townsend, in short, is most interested in water contamination and is attentive to sources of water and the effect of weather. A second, far more detailed map has differing geological areas bordered in six different colors and circles drawn over places showing registration data (see fig. 7.3). The circles act both as spots (that is, showing the location of disease) and as charts. Each circle is divided into quarters: the upper left half shows the date the first place was attacked, and the upper right half shows population per square mile. The lower left documents the percentage of villages attacked out of the total number of villages in the area and the lower right registers the percentage of mortality in the populations attacked. There are also dates written under some individual villages. A plain line is supposed to show places where cholera prevailed, but it is impossible to distinguish these from roads, which appear also to be shown. The map appears to be a topographic map, with data mapped onto it. The first map is apparently fulfilling the basic requirements of the report: to show the area affected and document some native activity to explain it; the second is a labor of love, created to advance an argument.

This map begins to do what other maps do not, that is, to treat India as a complex surface overlaying depths of variable materials; such a treatment

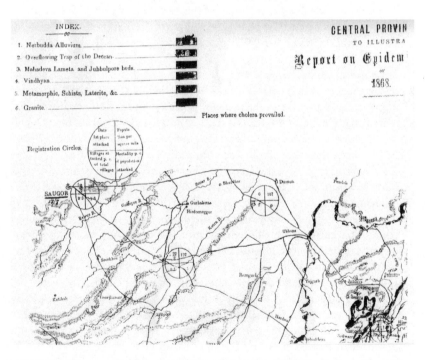

FIGURE 7.3. Townsend's Map: detail. From Townsend, Dr. S.C., Sanitary Commissioner, Central Provinces and Berars *Report on the Cholera Epidemic of 1868*. N.p.: n.p. 1869. Bound with Malleson and Cuningham. Image reproduced by permission of The Wellcome Library, London.

implies the possibility of melioration, as indeed do Townsend's detailed descriptions of the local soil and water supplies of individual villages. The map shows the major bodies of water and type of soil and stone underlying them, and relates the incidence of cholera to geological formation; Townsend uses the geological survey as bases for his own maps (85). This cross-referencing of maps which track different variables—here, the local geology—was essential to British mapping even by the late 1840s, and is necessary to the representation of the land as a complex and variable three-dimensional object subject to change. Its use for the first time to connect cholera mortality, a key index of social conditions, to these other variables in India suggests that the connection of the social body to a narrative of progress based on the transformation of the environment, so basic to nineteenth-century discourse on the metropole, is finally becoming thinkable by some British authorities in India.

CIVILIZATION AND BARBARISM: COMPARATIVE VISIONS OF SPACE

The 1860s had returned British medics to a wider global context, within which England and India are not wholly separate problems, but are located in a global continuum. Discussions of attempts to reinstitute modified cordons sanitaires, targeting especially Muslim pilgrims crossing the Red Sea, made international collaboration and British responsibility for communication between areas under their own administration and the larger world a necessary, if unpleasant object of contemplation, and the enormous increase of British troops, and thus also medics, in India following the Rebellion of 1857 also did much to bring the two medical literatures together by increasing contact between the two professional groups. Indian maps of the 1860s tend to assume some kind of human activity, and map that, as sanitary questions across larger India are less remediable than those of particular camps and fair locations, whereas maps of the 1860s in Britain are more concerned with specific sites and water supplies, which are seen as demanding identification and remediation.

Finally, the later maps of India are less preoccupied with epidemiological questions and more with administrative issues—how cholera got out of hand in a particular camp, and so forth. This is in part because its etiology was more clearly understood, but also, I suspect, in large part because responsibility for sanitary failures were squarely on colonial administrators' shoulders. British authorities, on the other hand, were certainly as interested in the occurrence of cholera in the Isles as ever, but they were also newly cognizant of being responsible for the pandemics. The Anglo-Indian sanitarian was responsible for his districts in India; the British government was responsible for the nation's relationship to the world. Further, the system of local sanitary authorities accompanying their reports with sanitary maps meant that there was a thorough and reasonably accurate, if stylistically inconsistent mapping of data in the Isles on a detailed scale which enabled the central government to turn its attention to larger issues. A large map literature not only fostered its own continuance, it provided a firm basis for the burgeoning of the study of epidemiological topography. The birth of tropical medicine as a specialty with claims to both professionalism and respectability is part of this outward looking movement and British mapping of itself into a larger and radically interconnected world.

The rhetoric of civilization and barbarism, culture and anarchy pervades the sanitary project as it does liberal discourse in general in this period. If lack of sanitation reveals a lingering barbarism in the heart of the civilized social body, wherein dirt is equated with viciousness and otherness, whether the otherness of the Irish slum dweller or the wealthy Briton who fails in Christian citizenship toward the larger community, the maps increasingly refine their search for this barbarism, seeking it in the hidden, below ground, and therefore past history of the city as the medical model gains on the sanitary vision of the visible, the apparent, the abject. On the one hand, this displaces authority and responsibility from the general community to a designated group of professionals who can surgically intervene in the body of the city. On the other, it displaces barbarism onto an inadequate history, a failing infrastructure redeemable in the interests of modernization, which becomes equal to civilization. Barbarism is figured as the degradation of the clean and proper body, the descent into a massed animalism expressed in poor sanitary and moral practices.

As we have said, Anglo-Indian contagionist (now including Snow adherents) medics' views received a boost from the Constantinople conference. The Conference's findings also put pressure on the British to manage the sanitary disaster of its Indian possessions. In the late 1860s, as we have seen, the need to exculpate themselves from responsibility for poor sanitation is quite evident in reports written by British sanitary authorities in India. One report begins by referring to the issue with entertaining candor: "With reference to paragraph 7 of Goverment Resolution No 398 of 1867, dated 25th February, 1867 ... I have the honour to submit the following report on the measures ... necessary to prevent Bombay being regarded by European nations as a base whence Cholera habitually spreads westward by the sea" (Hewlett 1). The report blames the spread of cholera on pilgrims from outside Bombay. Perhaps in part also for this reason, a small flurry of counterarguments did appear from insular medics clinging to meteorological and other explanations, and sometimes by refuting the claim that cholera had come from India. D. K. Whittaker, reporting for the *London Quarterly Review* on the cholera conference and recent cholera research, goes through an impressive number of historical documents in order to conclude that although cholera may be endemic to India, it does not necessarily emerge primarily from the Ganges valley. He remarks of the cholera conference's conclusions:

> It has been a favorite French notion to throw the onus of the production of cholera in India on English domination, and to attribute it to the neglect on the part of the English Government of the great canals and works of the Mohamedan emperors. This idea was broached before the Conference, but was entirely dissipated by our able English representatives. We need not inquire where those great works were situated, or at what period they fell into decay. It seems sufficient to remark, that cholera is first known to us in districts in which there never were such works, and that its great centre in India at present is in a part of India where none such ever existed. (22)

Although Whittaker nods to the importance of sanitation and drainage in the Ganges, he immediately turns to religious pilgrimmage both in India and to Mecca as the real target of concern (26–27), thus blaming cholera on the recalcitrant Indians rather than the land, which is a British possession.

One odd insular attempt to refute India as point of origin operated largely by simply never referring to it. Inspector General of Hospitals Robert Lawson's paper, "Further Observations on the Influence of Pandemic Waves in the Production of Fevers and Cholera," read March 2, 1868, was originally published in the *Transactions of the Epidemiological Society of London* and then reprinted in the 1880s as part of a larger volume in the Millbank lecture series, demonstrating that the paper enjoyed some popularity. The accompanying map shows a world defined by Asia in the east and the Americas in the west, with isoclinal lines showing "pandemic waves" moving from south to north.[4] Lawson's theory is based on a long-standing sense that cholera and "fever" were related (see fig. 7.4). "Fever" in the nineteenth century was an inclusive term from many febrile diseases, but was particularly associated with slum diseases such as typhus, smallpox, and typhoid. For many years, a substantial minority of medics claimed that cholera itself was a fever, despite its lack of febrile symptoms, and sanitarians pointed to its tendency to attack the same locations as fever. Lawson separates the two diseases, but retains the connection between the two. In his model, "Febrific" waves "move from South to North. They take five years to go from the Cape of Good Hope to England" (221). These waves, obviously, carry fever. "Cholerific" waves alternate with febrific waves, preceding and following them, as epidemic "fever" is thought to alternate with epidemic cholera. (It is perhaps worth noting that this period is approximately when the east-west dichotomy begins to give way to the south-north opposition, both in London and globally, as Africa moves toward center stage of the Empire.)

The stunning absence in Lawson's argument is any attempt to account for the clear history of evidence which placed India at the epicenter of the

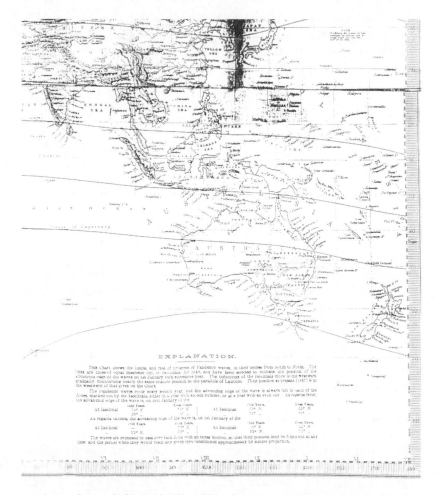

FIGURE 7.4. Lawson's Cholerific Wave Map. From Lawson, Robert. "Further Observations on the Influence of Pandemic Waves in the Production of Fevers and Cholera." read 2nd March, 1968, *Transactions of the Epidemiological Society of London,* Sessions 1866–1876. 3: 216–231.

disease, not to mention the more local medical topography of cholera epidemics, wherein its first entry into Britain in 1832 was at Sunderland—hardly the extreme south of the Isles—in the face of the Constantinople conference's much published findings. Perhaps it was attractive not only for its appeal to a meteorological and magnetic model, but also because it seemed to provide a way of declining responsibility for the spread of cholera.

Lawson's theory, despite its bizarre failure to mention India at all, echoes a larger controversy ongoing in British India after the conference. Despite the fact that English physicians had almost universally accepted the efficacy of sanitary measures, especially including the provision of clean water, whatever their reservations about the exact nature of cholera and its spread, a substantial minority of Indian medics—including, crucially, in Bengal, the acknowledged endemic center of cholera outbreaks—reverted to a climatic theory of cholera which, amazingly, was not only anticontagionist, but antisanitarian. W. R. Cornish complains that, "even in the present day so unsettled are the views of the profession that the old battle between the 'contagionists' and 'non-contagionists' bids fair to be fought over again with all its original fierceness" (1). This debate is best exemplified by the exchanges of this same Cornish, the contagionist medic of Madras, whose territory suffered successive invasions of cholera from Bengal, and Bryden, of Bengal, surgeon and statistical officer of the Sanitary Commission there. Bryden first published his views in the late 1860s that cholera was borne out of the endemic region into the epidemic ones on the monsoon winds, that it was noncontagious, that because it was native to part of Bengal and not related to sanitary conditions, sanitary measures would have no effect on it, that, in fact, it was a natural disaster beyond human control. As might be imagined, this conclusion, running counter to all conventional wisdom in Europe and most in India, and the findings of the International Sanitary Conference, raised eyebrows. In response, Bryden writes loftily:

> Those who can know little of the harmonies of epidemiology and of the rigid laws which govern these harmonies, would accuse me of sitting down with this vast collection of facts before me and ambitiously distorting each into a place in a system, which as a system has no real existence. Different observers will interpret the same facts differently. An uneducated man has no difficulty in satisfying himself that the ice-groovings on a boulder are the work of the stone-mason. In science, there is a recognizable limit to diversity of interpretation, and he whose education is the more complete can go further in advance of the man who has no intimate knowledge of the subject he professes to treat.
>
> It has been almost demanded that the result of a study of the cholera of India should show one immediately recognizable condition to be the cause of the outbreak. . . . When I have maintained that the epidemic is an inevitable evil . . . it has been asserted that such doctrines obstruct the progress of sanitation as a science. (*Epidemic* 2–3)

Bryden refers to the conference directly and refutes its findings. In the 1874 expanded version of his argument, he claims that Indian authorities have never ascribed to the contagionist views of the conference, quoting

Jameson and his followers at length, but failing to mention Scot or Cornish and Townsend, with whom, by then, he had had long and acrimonious disputes centered precisely around Scot's map (Bryden, *Cholera* 243–44). In this same 1874 document, he takes a stand for scientific objectivity against political pressures:

> The tendency of late years has been to study cholera more immediately in its relation to man, and to subordinate facts as they occur . . . to the theory of . . . the distribution of epidemic cholera by human intercourse, and of its multiplication in the human economy but nobody in India really accepts that explanation, and were we now to accept it . . . it cannot be doubted that the progress of the study of cholera on a true because on a natural basis, would be indefinitely retarded. The present is an opportune occasion for re-opening this question on a basis of statistical facts. (*Cholera* 2)

Bryden also refers to the attraction which plans to quarantine Bengal have for many people, but asserts that such a step would make no difference to the spread of disease (*Epidemic* 2). In short, the demands of the International Sanitary Conference split British medics into two camps, one which basically agreed with the general consensus in Europe, and one which was decidedly reactionary. The disagreement between these two groups would propel British medical mapping in India into a new phase.

Surgeon W. R. Cornish of Madras was appalled and infuriated by Bryden's argument, the more so since his own region was regularly invaded. Countering Bryden and his use of Jameson, Cornish draws upon the mapping of his own area by Scot, who had been as contagionist as Jameson was anti. Cornish is clear that the cholera is Bryden's problem: "[M]alignant or epidemic cholera is not a natural product of Southern India"; instead it invades from the north:

> [W]e have been in the habit of supposing that the disease was a true endemic of the soil [in some of southern India where it lingered for three or four years]; but, although the conditions of the soil and climate in such districts probably approach very nearly to the conditions of the natural habitat of cholera in Lower Bengal, yet there are probably some points of difference as yet unascertained. (2)

And again, Cornish stresses that in his district, "[c]holera is like a foreign plant in them, that has found a fairly congenial, but not wholly natural soil, so that after a certain definite time the plant dies" (3). He then quotes Scot verbatim at length, asserting that subsequent epidemics have all followed the same route, and pointedly asserts that Scot's work is "all the more valuable at the present time, because it was compiled not to illustrate any 'theory' of invasion, but to record, in a connected form, the testimony of officers of the Medical Department, who had personally witnessed the outbreak" (14). He explains that he has "redrawn" Scot's map (in fact, drawn by V. Vardaraja Moodely, facing page 15), and has added several arrows to show the direction of the monsoon winds, both from the southwest and the northeast (see fig. 7.5). Unfortunately, he has also removed the marked roads, which in Scot's map so clearly showed human carriage; the topographic detail of mountains is also missing.

Cornish then launches into an indignant refutation of Bryden, whose maps, he states, are "wholly misleading":

> [I]f we are to trust to Dr. Bryden's figures and maps, the invading cholera of that year stopped short in what he calls the 'eastern division of the epidemic area,' viz, the districts eastward of Gwalior, Saugor, and Jubbulpore. . . . It is somewhat strange that a cholera map should have been drawn for 1859 so as

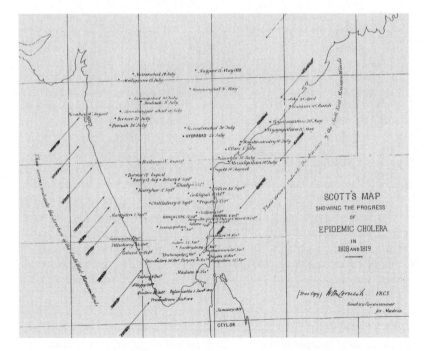

FIGURE 7.5. Cornish's Redrawing of Scot's Map with Arrows showing Monsoon Wind Direction: detail. From Cornish, W.R., *Report on Cholera in Southern India for the Year 1869, with map illustrative of the disease.* Madras: H. Morgan, 1870.

to show a complete exemption of the western and southern tracts, the more
especially as it is evident from the report that Dr. Bryden was acquainted
with the fact of the invasion of Bombay in that year. (15)

Cornish repeats his version of Bryden's maps (seven times, each showing a different time period) and extends them to show the south and the geography
and temporality of epidemic invasion there—incidentally, by repeating them,
he reiterates the endemicity of the northeast (see fig. 7.6). Cornish's arguments have not changed since his earlier report: pilgrims and coolies spread
cholera, and he finds Bryden's casual dismissal of Hurdwar pilgrims as vectors
monstrous. The keynote of his argument, however, is his reproduction of
Scot's map, with the addition of arrows showing wind direction during the
monsoons, which, he argues, shows clearly that the monsoons do not spread
cholera (78). He insists that every epidemic has followed the same path since
Scot charted the first one.

Cornish is basically happy with the condition of Madras, reiterating that
it is pilgrims who spread disease:

> [S]imple sanitary precautions should be enforced, at all times, with the class
> of people who constitute the bulk of pilgrim visitors to celebrated shrines,
> but it does not help forward the progress of sanitary science to credit
> attempts at enforcement of cleanliness and decency, with the power of avert-
> ing an advancing wave of cholera. . . . The intensity of cholera, and the pro-
> longation of its epidemic visitations, are, I am convinced, largely due to the
> habits of the people in gadding about to divers places where festivals are
> held, and their unnatural modes of living during such seasons. (149–50)

However, Cornish argues, against Bryden's total disregard of sanitary
improvement as useless, that such improvement does make a material difference, observing dryly that if Bengal cannot be improved vis-à-vis sanitation,
it must be a very different place than it was a few years earlier, when the 1861
Cholera Commission found its sanitary conditions wanting (151). He concludes, pointedly, that he trusts that soon "a systematic effort to attack and
defeat cholera in its endemic home, shall be made with every prospect of
modifying those periodical invasions of epidemics which now carry terror and
dismay, and destruction of life, over nine-tenths of the habitable globe"
(160)—including his own innocent corner of it.

Cornish was not the most eloquent defender of the faith, and his waffling
on the topic of sanitary improvements—Madras doesn't need them, but Bengal does—did not help him much. Bryden rose, exultant, to the challenge,
reproducing Cornish's reproduction of Scot's map and, adding several lines
denoting areas of successive epidemic invasion, manages through a rather
spectacular manipulation of data to adduce Scot's map as evidence for his own

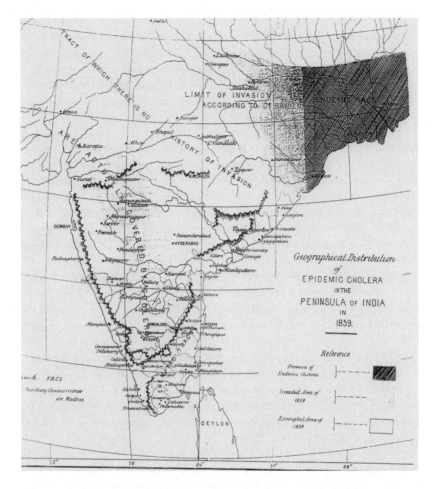

FIGURE 7.6. Cornish's Reprint of Bryden's map with Added Material: detail. From Cornish, W.R., *Report on Cholera in Southern India for the Year 1869, with map illustrative of the disease.* Madras: H. Morgan, 1870.

theory: "In [Scot's] map, I have inserted in the North, stations where Jameson's record tells us were first invaded in May 1818. . . . This cholera, had a definite boundary line in the South, which I have dotted in on Scott's map [. . .] demarcations shown between May and July 1818" (*Epidemic* 6n) and likewise between July and August, and August and October, which, according to Bryden, showed cholera's advance "per saltum"—that is, in leaps covering simultaneously an entire region affected by monsoon winds. He exults in the happiness of having more data to fill out his theory and chides his predecessors, "Records of the epidemic intervening are made up of fragmentary data which were never placed in order to form a consistent history, probably because it was deemed impossible that a connected history of cholera could be written for any year or any epidemic, although the simple narration of Scott and Jameson now show us that all through these fifty years an accurate and connected record might have been kept up" (*Epidemic* 2n).

Future splutterings by Cornish and others were grandly ignored. It is hard, from the vantage point of the present, not to indict Bryden for a callous, cynical and self-serving misuse of evidence in the interest of exculpating the Bengal authorities from responsibility, both for past epidemics and for any sanitary improvement. His arrogant dismissal of his critics as "uneducated" doesn't make him any more likeable. However, it is also important to keep in mind that medics living in the endemic area may have experienced it very differently than those living outside those regions. Bryden, Jameson's regional heir, shares many of his views, and that may be because their experiences were similar. However, where Jameson blamed Indian practices for sanitary problems and recommended increasing drainage, sewerage and the like, Bryden shifts all the blame to the landscape, exonerating the government from any attempt to solve the problem. Notably, in his many citations of Jameson, he fails to mention these recommendations. Further, it is difficult not to hold Bryden, with the experience of other medics all over the world to draw on, to a higher standard of the openness he so ostentatiously claims. In answering critics who wondered why measures which had worked in Europe wouldn't be useful in India, he responded, simply, "[O]n the ground of homology, I am prepared to believe that the aspect of cholera in Europe may be very different from that presented to our study in India. As I remarked in my original report—'The relative value of the primary and secondary truths probably differs much in different countries and among different races'" (*Cholera* 40).

It should also be said that in 1868, Malleson and Cuningham's formal *Report on the Cholera* for the same area politely disagreed with Bryden (136), and advocated both for sanitary reforms and human carriage of the disease, as discussed above. By 1873, however, Cuningham is using a map which is based on Bryden's, and is anticontagionist to the point of arguing that pilgrims are not particularly subject to the disease (15–17). While still sanitarian, he also dismisses water contamination as a cause (20–25). Like Bryden, Cuningham insists his observations are only good for the cholera in India (32), thus undoing the work of his forebears in the first decade of the nineteenth century and the 1830s who attempted to interest insular readers on the strengths of the cholera's similarity of functioning in India and Europe. Unlike Bryden, however, he is anxious to avoid controversy, pleading that he is only contributing to the sum total of facts which will one day unravel the cholera mystery (32).

What must interest us about this spat, in addition to its illustration of the tendencies of medical theories to follow local political interests, is that it sparked the first detailed historical analyses of cholera epidemics and use of multiple maps to reinvest the epidemics with a sense of historical narrative. Bryden (and later Cuningham) uses few maps, preferring charts, and all his care is directed to a story of a timeless cycle—a homogenous land visited by an annual cycle of monsoons which must always have the same result. His narrative is a narrative of inevitable repetition, a land caught in time. He is thus in direct opposition to his contemporaries in Britain in his portrayal of disease and geography. His maps tend to strip the land of its features, including mountains, rivers, roads, and so forth, since those are extraneous to his argument and also suggest other possible theses. However, in giving the disease a history and a narrative extending backward in time and space, he opens the door for Cornish, however blunderingly, to use his maps to show several different trajectories of the epidemic in successive years. Despite his claim that the cholera always follows generally the same path, his maps tell us that there are many variations in the path of the disease, just as his narrative focuses on the possibility of melioration through sanitation and possibly quarantine of pilgrims, a notion dear to Cornish's heart.

Despite Bryden's call for a continuous narrative, then, it is Cornish who actually gives us a narrative—that is, a sequence of events defined by change—despite the fact that both men's ideological blind spots lead them to insist that cholera is always the same! Townsend, who appears to have teamed up with Cornish to question Bryden's results, of course, had long been interested in a vision of an India subject to progress through drainage. It is in the 1860s, then, that we begin to see a concerted drift among some medics and other mappers toward a layered, historically more nuanced vision of India's land.[5] This, of course, may be partially related to the rise of Orientalist study which was related to political management, and I don't want simply to glamorize it as antiracist or anti-imperialist. However, the emergence of this trend did enable a vision of Indian land to emerge in the British imaginary which could be emplaced in a narrative of progress and change—and, perhaps, a vision of India which suggested the possibility of a history which extended beyond the boundaries of British occupation, both backwards and forward in time.

Finally, though Bryden's motives must remain obscure, it is certainly clear that the effect of his fatalistic arguments were to excuse the British government in Bengal from making any efforts toward melioration at all; a furious Cornish and Townsend repeatedly demanded inquiries into Bryden's investigations, but Bryden did not budge an inch, was promoted to surgeon major, and four years after the initial publication of his thesis, brought out the definitive and greatly expanded version of the same argument, analysing several years of data, to arrive at exactly the same conclusion. Of course, his voice was one among many, and was not definitive in policymaking. It is ironic that, whereas insular mappers finally used early Anglo-Indian maps to construct a more nuanced view of the cholera in England, after years of neglect, Indian mappers never did use maps historically until after the International Sanitary Conference, when medics such as Bryden were insistent on the nontransferability of knowledge from India to Europe. Detailed historical cholera mapping in India didn't really take off until Bryden had provoked resistance which turned to the techniques of English mappers to refute him. Snow may never have been able to develop his theory without recourse to the Indian materials; that alone makes their inclusion in English medical history significant. In turn, ironically, it is the English tradition which finally gives Anglo-Indian mappers, belatedly, a way to begin to narrate India as site with a history of its own.

CONCLUSION

As we have seen, disease mapping in India was pursued energetically at the same time as it was in Europe. However, maps from India were largely ignored by insular medics in the 1830s. There are a number of reasons for this. The contagionist model that tended to dominate these maps was not welcome in a country opposed to quarantines for economic reasons. British medics in the 1830s were inclined to disbelieve that this was the same disease that had ravaged India for some years. "Why now? Why here?" they asked. But there was also a kind of double marginalization of the other: India, a land caught in the past, a static or degenerating "old" society simply could not be experiencing the same epidemic as a land so far distanced in space and time. Further, the medics who worked in India may have lacked the cultural authority with their insular peers for their maps to have the same ability to assert truth claims. Expatriate medics complain bitterly of being ignored and ridiculed in the insular medical press and also of being accused of arrogance when they stood upon their considerable field experience in contrast to the insular lack of contact with the disease. Also these were largely surgeons in an era when physicians and theoretic knowledge ruled over experience and surgical authority.

Later, when it became undeniable that this was the same epidemic, and when relations between physicians and surgeons, between theoretic and field knowledge, were beginning to reverse, many insular medics (with the pointed exception of Snow and Farr) still largely ignored their colleagues in South Asia, in part because of theories of racial difference beginning to gain ground in the late 1850s and early 1860s, but perhaps also in part because of real differences in the mapping traditions. It is interesting to note the differences in the construction of the two objects of study in maps made by Britons and readily available in Britain, in part because the techniques used for both began as similar practices and diverged so widely.

Indian maps, like British maps, began in the 1820s and 1830s as large-scale representations of the continent or region and the isle respectively. In general, as we have seen, Indian maps showed a stronger tradition of contagionism. In part, this was simply a matter of scale. One-to-one spot maps of deaths, even could they have been made, would have been a meaningless pointillist blur in a map of, say, all of the northern Indian territory. Information regarding morbidity was uncertain, and tended to be richest in areas the British travelled frequently, and among the British and their troops themselves. Early in the century, detailed, accurate maps of India (according to British standards) were still difficult to come by, and there is some evidence that even the use of the graticule was more a decorative convention than a sign of proper scaling (see Edney 321). India maps, therefore, are often regional maps organized by lines of spread, which tend to be represented as following waterways and roads. In part because the British despaired of correcting the sanitation of such a large and populous territory, in part because of the expense, and in part because of racist assumptions that Indians were naturally dirty and therefore that cholera was a part of their natural habitat (see Prashad), Britons at midcentury rarely micromapped the Indian territories either, despite a radical improvement in the availability of topographically accurate maps. Detailed mappings from in the 1860s tend to be of Anglo settlements (carefully separated from their neighboring Indian towns) or of temporary sites built by the British in which cholera attacked—military camps and festival sites for religious pilgrims. In these sites, what Britons saw as the deleterious nature of India itself or the equally deleterious habits (generally connected to religion) of the people were cited as causes which could not be remedied.

In this way, abstract space in India was not at this time, as it was in London, the space of the palimpsest. Unlike England, where the landscape had layers which were defective but meliorable, India was not susceptible of improvement. The land of India itself was seen as guilty of disease production. Whereas low lying, damp areas in England were seen as unhealthy and vulnerable to colonization by disease until drained, India, and the people and behaviors that were mapped onto the land, were considered to constitute an ecological entity productive of evil. David Arnold has also observed the increasing tendency in the first half of the century of Britons to imagine the entire diverse geography of India as homogenously tropical *(Problem of Nature)*, and the tropics themselves represented a sullied Eden, a condition of humanity simultaneously childlike and degenerate (see, for example Kingsley or Tennyson. In fact, about half of India sits above the tropic of Cancer.)

Although medics speak of the sedimentation of a very old culture being the very source of cholera, that sedimentation is not seen as layers of change in a country moving toward modernity, as it is in England. Instead, it is simply the sedimentation of a stagnant culture caught endlessly in a single moment of past time—a time of barbarism.

When India is seen as having degenerated from a past glory, at some point in the distant past, this progression or regression is presented as having stopped. Micromapping is not necessary because there are no distinctions in the layers. The level of the graticule is the appropriate level of abstraction for the imposition of a British logic and British settlements, at an appropriate distance, from the monstrous and monumental barbarism of India. Although this was undoubtedly often not the intention, or even the perception, of the mapmakers, other factors, often economic and political, contributed to a representation of India that depended on and perpetuated this perception. Those Britons who objected to this view—and there were many—were largely ignored, as were the natives who lobbied for such assistance. While English visions of space became increasingly layered, susceptible of what I have termed a "realist" narration of progress and the structural equivalence of bodies, representations of Indian space became ever more solidly "mythic" tending toward narrative embedded in static or cyclical time and embodying fixed characteristics.

Mapping in India, then, did not tend to the level of abstraction in representation that British insular mapping could sometimes achieve. Cartograms of London sometimes relied on the viewer's knowledge of the terrain to minimize geographic information in favor of maximizing the kind of detailed data that could best be given in a chart, thus combining some of the elements of both charts and maps, as in chapter 3, fig. 3.7, a cartogram that situates place-names roughly in proper spatial relation to each other and to a Thames river that is simplified into a straight line separating north from south. The use of charts in combination with maps is comparatively rare in Indian maps, whereas basic geographic data (the shape of the continent, the parallels, and so on) are almost never absent. Micromapping and audience familiarity with the object of representation allow for multiple views of, say, London in a way they simply don't for India.[6]

This "denial of coevalness" as Johannes Fabian would put it—the distancing of another in space and time which simultaneously legitimates the scientific gaze and neutralizes difference by casting it in the distant developmental past in relation to the observer—obviously has its appeal, from a simply economic and administrative standpoint. Sanitizing India would have been expensive; if India was, however, by its essential nature unsanitary, then it was impossible to expect British administration to have much impact on it. As Prashad writes, "India (they) acts as a metaphor for all that the European (we) is not. What *they* are, fits for *them*, since it is the natural environment which *they* need 'in order to prosper.' [For them the] filth is not filth" (256). Projected onto the landscape, this filthy body, improperly contained, without clear boundaries, is the direct opposite of the clearly defined, modern urban body which underlay the public health projects of the metropole.

This attitude made it possible to leave Indians in the Augean stables which imperialism had helped create but which, in the perception of many British, was simply an unalterable part of the Indian landscape. It also made it possible to ignore that in fact India had changed a good deal in the nineteenth century, what with massive British public works projects which, recent scholarship suggests, had a role in causing endemic cholera to get out of hand (David Arnold, *Problem*). But such representations, however cynically adumbrated they may have been in some cases, contributed to the general perception of the Orient as the West's other and the consolidation of images of the liberal Western self in the metropole as individual, secular, bourgeois, scientific, modern, and capable of being imaged harmoniously at both the micro and macro level, as bodies literally permeated with information which was available and generalizable at several levels of abstraction. The other, however, was the dense, massive, unknowable body of barbaric people who resisted visibility and penetration by grids of information. The land could be controlled at the level of the graticule; the people were passively sedimented onto that land and incapable of the civilization, the transparency, the modernity that susceptibility to micromapping implied. Perhaps, then, Indian disease maps were so long ignored because of the British sense of the inevitability of cholera in that context, as opposed to their commitment to its evitability in modern Britain. The Other was trapped, like a fly in amber, in one layer and moment of a time long past.

The International Sanitary Conference of 1866 prompted a number of policy measures, mostly quarantining of religious pilgrims and so forth, and finally toward the end of the century, more attention to sanitation. But the development of medical mapping in England and India to midcentury—a development, especially in the case of cholera, which sets up a mutually defining relationship based on difference between the two—dovetails with liberal understanding of the social body and midcentury racial ideology to produce a vision of Britain based on a layered body developing toward modernity. In this body, atavism or degeneration can be found and fixed in the earlier layers of an increasingly civilized body, city, self—a vision against which could be positioned a view of the colonial other as a nonlayered, unalterable subject and landscape whose surface and depth were likewise frozen in time, a subject without interiority. In an era in which proper compliance with sanitation equalled civilization and readiness for citizenship, John Stuart Mills excluded, in speaking of India as an immature culture, non-European cultures from readiness for even the access to those rights which were thought to develop such values, as Uday Singh Mehta points out. Positioning India as both child and senescent culture, both before the present of Britain developmentally and as a past civilization in historical terms, allowed Indians to be positioned outside of liberal universalism, which posited a complex subject in whom present and past were simultaneously contained—a representation which was linked to representations of Indian geography. At last, in the late 1860s, British medics in India begin to be able to map the country as a land with a medical history—and perhaps a future.

AFTERWORD

Still Visible Today

The best performance in the fantoccini is that of the figure which, in the act of dancing, becomes disjointed yet every joint, still pregnant with vitality, continues to dance as gaily as ever. . . . So long as the machinery is perfect, and the performer sober, all goes well; but if the main string should break, the figure would fall in a disjointed wreck. . . . The metropolis is very like that figure. When we first view it as a whole, it appears to be complete and closely knit, and its actions are energetic if not graceful. If we continue to observe we see in due time that its several limbs or component parts are easily separated, that after separation they are still vital and active, generally speaking more active than before, and so the dance goes on quite gaily. But if the string should break that ties the whole together! Awful thought, that a social chaos must be the consequence. . . . [I]t is worn to a thread, it does not act its part with integrity, and here and there a limb separated from the rest, and, energetically kicking, refuses to glide back to its place in the metropolitan anatomy. If we could get the figure to stand still for a moment, we should behold it in its perfection, but, unhappily, it is full of life, and that, so to speak, is death for it, for the limbs will get away from the trunk.

—"Metropolitan Confusions," the *City Press,* 1866

No one knows for sure just how AIDS began. The first people to get sick with AIDS were in central Africa. Most people think it must have started in that part of the world. Now it is all over the world.

—Anna Forbes, *Where Did AIDS Come From?*

187

BY THE END OF THE CENTURY, medical mapping was fully integrated into public health discourse and was increasingly standardized. The confusion and multiplicity that reigned earlier dissipated, and with it, the potential for dramatic new changes in the public imagination of community. However, the earlier impact of such mapping lingered in other forms; perhaps its influence is seen most clearly in late modern views of the city as a body. We have seen how sanitary and medical mapping functioned within both a professional and juridical setting to legitimate certain definitions of community, and to transform the gaze of the urban administrator into one determined by spatial and medical parameters. We have also noted how such visions of the city intertwined with, coopted, or were resisted by urban mapping schema "on the ground" of inhabitants, other professionals, and so on. Now I would like to briefly sketch out how such visions of the city affected the shape of nineteenth- and twentieth-century urbanism itself—its theories of urban growth, its concepts of urban management in the nineteenth century—and to trace some of the legacies of discourse that have persisted in the urban imaginary into the present day.

We have seen how first sanitary maps, such as Gavin's, and then medical maps, such as Snow's, laid out a vision of London as a body. Over the second half of the nineteenth century, cautious optimism about London as an organic body whose systems could be made visible through mapping and subject to medical intervention balanced with anxiety about the monstrous size and uncontrolled growth of London the leviathan. Untrammeled growth—the cancerous city—could also be read as inherently unhealthy, incapable of containment and thus improvement and modernity. Circulatory connections that made the city powerful also made it vulnerable, as Snow demonstrated. This understanding became foundational to the much better known late-nineteenth-century poverty maps and urban theory of Charles Booth. Booth, in turn, serves as a bridge between the mid-nineteenth century and our own time, leading toward some recent voices in urban planning. Some urban planning today still retains an unacknowledged, because unconscious, connection to assumptions about the city rooted in nineteenth-century public health mappings.

BOOTH AND LONDON'S BODY

The most famous thematic maps of London are undoubtedly those of the late-nineteenth-century Booth project. The *Pall Mall Gazette* hailed Booth as a "social copernicus" *[sic]* whose recentering of the metropolitan universe was understood to have profound effects on the understanding of the social body of London. This massive undertaking sought to map many behaviors and aspects of life in London, but most crucially, it mapped poverty, street by street and often house by house. Using seven colors to distinguish levels of affluence, Booth coded wealth as warm and light (yellow representing the wealthy and red the well-off) down through successive shades of cooler colors (pink, purple, light blue) to the very poor (dark blue), with the "vicious, criminal" level of poverty in the night shade of black. In this sense, he built on the tradition of nineteenth-century iconography and also the convention of conversion of economic into moral status, particularly at the lower reaches of the scale.

Like Snow's map, Booth's maps also enabled viewers to see the city as an organic and connected whole: unlike any map which came earlier, they worked at such a sophisticated level of particularity that it became possible to trace the trajectory of the spatial development and movement of affluence over time. It became apparent to Booth that the city developed in rings of population and that in older industrial sections where population was concentrated, poverty was sure to be found. His maps also displayed the proximate relationship between wealth and poverty, the wealth to the northwest of the Thames depending on the poverty of the north; the comfort of the middle classes throughout the west and central areas dependent on the poverty to the south and east. Most tellingly, Booth's maps made visual knowledge of what had been long folkloric wisdom: that although extreme wealth clustered together, the upper middle class lined the fronts of large streets which backed onto and turned into side streets and courts of decreasing affluence. In short, it made the point that behind the large thoroughfare down which middle-class readers habitually walked or rode, with its evident display of health and comfort, there existed a thinly veiled reality of less fortunate, less healthy bodies upon which the display of affluence rested.

The face of London was deceptive: mapping laid open the corrupt body beneath the facade and could also begin to expose the laws by which it degenerated. The booming, buzzing confusion of London could be made legible by observing the shifts and gradations of color. As on an anatomical slide, the color of the stain revealed the nature of the tissue under the gaze of the scientist. Within this organic metaphor is included a corporeal model of circulation. It is clear that the middle classes represent the healthy tissue, the economic lifeblood of the city, the vibrant red following the major thoroughfares of the metropolis, backed by pink and lavender. Pockets of corruption, however, are vividly picked out in the colors of death. Seen overall, the west appears to be a healthy, bright orange-red with pockets of darkness. The east, however, and to some extent the south, range from a pallidly underoxegenated pinkish-lavender to a chilling pale blue, with threateningly concentrated blotches of dark blue and black (see fig. A.1). Given the ethnic distribution of the London population, this darkness takes on racial overtones as well.

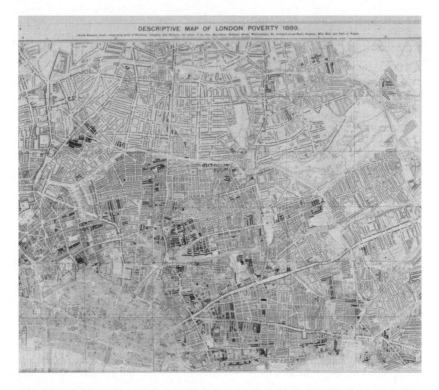

FIGURE A.1. Booth Poverty Map, N.E. London: detail. From Booth, Charles, ed. *Life and Labour of the People in London.* 9 vols. London: Macmillan and Co., 1897.

David Reeder provides an excellent analysis of Booth's work, arguing that "the whole point . . . was to reveal the regularities in the metropolitan condition, to expose its orderliness, and thus to make London comprehensible" (325). As Reeder observes, Booth is attentive to the movements of wealth and fascinated by what seem to operate as rules for the distribution in space of a particular class. Reeder remarks that Booth accounts for the preponderance of wealthy in certain neighborhoods by noting the desire of the well-to-do to live on higher ground, and the tendency of areas which were cut off from major thoroughfares or which were cul de sacs susceptible of entry from only one direction to be inhabited by the poor (330). Reeder goes on to note that this is part of Booth's "evolutionary and residualist" understanding of poverty, such areas forming a "sump or settlement tank into which the detritus of the metropolis is poured" (332).

Reeder's metaphor, in part taken from Booth's, is more telling than perhaps he realizes. Booth's understanding of poverty is profoundly informed by nineteenth-century sanitary and medical understandings of both public and individual health. Wealthy people did seek high ground, in part because it was, for at least half a century, believed to be healthier than the low terrain. Booth thus comes to his hypothesis through analysis of a medical understanding he shares with his subjects. His dislike of enclosed spaces also relates to sanitary science—enclosed spaces were thought to be dark and airless (a belief which is reflected in the anoxic tints of such sites on the map itself). But perhaps most crucially, we see again the notion of circulation encoded in the anatomical representation of London's body. These enclosed spaces are not connected to the circulatory vessels of the city; starved for the circulation, both physically, of healthy air and water, and economically, of capital and labor, such areas wither and die, rotting and then corrupting the urban social body.

Although somewhat attentive to differences between poor areas in his prose, Booth's color scheme homogenizes the poor. As David Englander points out, often areas were given economic categories based on the inhabitants' behavior: one street was "changed from dark to light blue" because police reported that it was "not troublesome" (322), and Jewish immigrants, having social characteristics associated with several different classes of English (for example, personally clean but not conventionally "house-proud"), puzzled Booth's inspectors when they tried to assign a color to their neighborhoods (306–307). Thus, Booth's supposedly rigorously economic taxonomy was in large part actually based on the traditional categories of domestic and social behavior that had informed the mid-Victorian sanitary movement. It is not surprising, then, that both the iconography of Booth's map and (one might say therefore) the spatial and representational logic of his interpretations are founded on the kind of anatomical vision of the city as a body so powerfully instantiated in Snow's work, and on the connection of poverty and disease to immorality and domestic slovenliness inscribed by sanitarians like Gavin.

Booth's ambivalent attempt to measure economic health divorced from the social highlights a central problem of late Victorian liberalism, its contradictory affirmation of individualism and distrust of the mass, and its foundational assumption of economic interdependence. He remarks, "When great aggregations of population are brought together, there is . . . a tendency toward uniformity of class in each section" (*Charles* 313). Such poverty arises from "[t]he thousand opportunities for earning precarious livelihoods presented by great centres of population" (*Charles* 303), but it also arises from the fact that the metropolis is not a center of large-scale production, as Booth recognizes. In lamenting that large factories are mostly choosing to locate in the provinces, Booth remarks that London compensates with small workshops and sweating systems which are "socially bad but economically advantageous," leading to irregular employment, long hours and low wages (*Charles* 110).

Booth is caught. On the one hand, he must acknowledge that these shops are "socially bad"—difficult for a proponent of laissez-faire. On the other hand, while he admires their economic "fitness" in one sentence, in a passage only a page or so away, he refers to these East London trades as "a clear case of economic disease" (*Charles* 109). While the poverty of the East London worker is exacerbated by foreign competition and that of women home workers, the real death blow is dealt by provincial British manufactory. The solution? Population must "adjust itself to the facts" and disperse to the new boom towns (*Charles* 110). In other words, the solution to the metropolis is to reduce its size.

Booth's understanding of the movement of population defined London as inhabited by concentric and centrifugal demographic rings:

> [F]orces . . . through increased pressure at the center . . . tend to drive or draw the resident population outwards in every direction. . . . [G]enerally the movement takes place gradually, from ring to ring, accompanied by a slow change of class. But the advance on new grounds shows a noticeable tendency to shoot out tongues, like the sun's corona. . . . These tongues follow the "lie of the land" and the facilities offered for speculation in building; but the more important cause . . . is always found in the available means of communication. (*Charles* 329)

Booth recommends a full-scale project to promote "improved means of communication," which also stands for transport, noting that, although some may worry that this will foster even more centralization, he believes it will have the opposite effect; small town centers will spring up in outlying areas (*Charles* 330). He calls for careful urban planning to avoid untrammeled building which would lead to congestion in favor of a more even distribution, with full communication, through roads and railways, to all parts of the urban corpus.

In effect, Booth's vision of the metropolis as a monstrous organism which has outgrown its inadequate circulatory system leads him to a distrust of a city large enough to have a true urban core: such a size leads inevitably to decay and corruption, skyrocketing land prices and overcrowding. In response to this, Booth recommends decentralization and a focus on "local life," the unreasoning and sick mass of the overgrown social body to be broken into its constituent parts. This formulation, both of urban development and decay proceeding in rings and of the healthiness of an unimpeded flow of labor and goods through the circulatory system of multiple bodies unified by a single communication system, has continued to be foundational to urban planning for the past century. It also still often takes its metaphoric base from the model of the city as an organic and unified body, and the metropolis as a cancerous overgrowth of the same.

There is a clear ambivalence in Booth's celebration of London—"our Jerusalem" (*Charles* 339)—and his fear of its massiveness. Again and again, Booth's nineteenth-century liberal vision is evident in his distrust of the massive or uniform, and celebration of individualism and the domestic virtues. Exasperated, he ends his "Housing" chapter in the "Recommendations"section by remarking, "I wish I could rouse in the minds of speculative builders a sense of the money value that lies in individuality, with its power of attracting the eye, rooting the affections, and arousing pride in house and home" (*Charles* 326). On the other hand, the metropolis is a necessary Darwinian crucible for the "new" England:

> Closely connected with the vitality and expansion of industry, we trace the advancement of the individual which in the aggregate is represented by the vitality and expansion of London. This is it that draws from the Provinces their best blood, and amongst Londoners selects the most fit . . . [characterized by upward mobility]. A new middle class is thus forming, which will, perhaps, hold the future in its grasp. . . . To them . . . political power will pass. (*Charles* 334)

According to H. Llewelyn Smith, writing for Charles Booth, "healthy" London is a hungry organism comprised of British, and mostly English provincials: "London is to a great extent nourished by the literal consumption of bone and sinew from the country" (in Booth *Life* 1: 508). Impoverished East London, however, as yet another map graphically shows, is largely comprised of two groups: foreigners and native born Londoners. Since native Londoners are degenerate (the city causes good stock to decay in three generations), native Londoners are not desirable. Ernest Aves, also writing for Booth, cites as a "natural disadvantage" of London "the physical deterioration of Londoners" (*Life* 9: 183). The "good" resident soon moves out toward the periphery; those who remain weaken and die out.

London, thus, is a great beast which devours the best and brightest who are drawn in and fail to escape. "The Circe among cities," London "too often exercises over her visitants her irresistible fascination only in the end to turn them into swine" (*Life* 1: 554). The good thing, however, about the London crucible, are those who do leave. Charles Booth, waffling between this almost wholly antiurban stance and admiration for the metropolis as crucible of healthy competition—amends Llewelyn Smith's report, adding,

> Population flows out of, as well as into, the great cities, so that the movement, looked at nationally, is a circulation, which is not only healthy in itself, but essential to national health. It may be too much to say that this circulation is caused by the deteriorating influence of city life, but the connection between the two is very close. To complain that men living in towns

degenerate physically is almost like complaining that the blood loses its oxygen in passing through our veins. Movements of population—interchange between town and country, or between centre and extremities—are of the very essence of civilization: the word implies as much: and of these movements that between London and the provinces is the most notable example. The mischief springs from the deposit which the stream of life leaves as it flows in country, no doubt, as well as in town. (Booth *Life* 1: 556)

Behind the healthy artery of circulation lies anoxic capillaries clogged with the detritus of those bodies, like Dickens's Jo, who dies when he can no longer "move on." To this end, Booth hopes for an increase in the promotion of a decentralized "individual responsibility." The mighty organism must be resolved into its component bodies; that disconnection will eliminate both social decay and the perils of contagion.

In this way, Booth recommends a decentered suburban ideal wherein both consumption and political identity revolve around the home: "Wherever a man may go to find his work, it is near home that he will seek his pleasure, and his wife will find her shopping . . . with brilliant shops, streets full of people, churches, and chapels certainly, perhaps a Town Hall, and probably a theater" (*Charles* 330). These aspects of life can be separated from production ("Wherever a man may . . . find his work"). Thus the economic productivity affiliated with a great metropolis can be retained, while the dangers of its massive social body can be avoided by the creation of independent local social and political bodies based on consumption. (How this relates to his earlier observation that trade is leaving the metropolis for the provinces is unclear.) Economic interdependence becomes the principle of communication within the metropole, but Booth retreats to individualism and local identity to avoid confronting the horror of the urban social body as a mass. The visibility of the city through mapping, so often figured as a means toward perfect modernity, highlights instead the inherently perverse vitality of the city at the expense of its enervated inhabitants; what becomes visible, finally, is modernity as monstrosity. Village England, surrounding a modern metropolis in which no one actually lives, becomes a way to recoup the promise of the modern city (individuality, transparency, freedom) without its pains through a nostalgic recourse to an ersatz past.

Whereas Gavin had noted the isolation of specific communities as cause for alarm in a radically interconnected urban body, Booth retreats to a suburban separatism to contain the cancerous spread of untrammelled growth. He carefully separates the economic body—a body that should operate on laissez-faire principles enhanced by a free and open circulation system—from the political and social body which must be planned, groomed, and maintained in cellular units. Ironically, these highly "individualized" cells are all to follow the same model: a town hall, a theater, a center of consumption. Booth, well intentioned and deeply concerned about the high level of impoverishment, is finally limited by his liberalism. His vision both pays homage to Gavin and Snow's emerging understanding of the urban body's permeability—the radical connectedness of economic and social factors and its relation to health—and refuses that organic unity, attempting to cordon off that circulation by breaking down the city into homogenous and manageable units based on the bourgeois domestic individualism so often proposed as a liberal response to the culture and economy of poverty. The final disavowal of the coterminous nature of the economic and the social body fails to resolve the problems highlighted by the last thirty years of social analysis in England: that poverty produces disease and vice, rather than the other way around, and that metropolitan capitalism requires poverty, both local and peripheral, as a resource. Perhaps we can see here a dim foreshadowing of the ability of global capitalism to cloak the nature of its operations in a superficial demarcation of local markets and celebration of their "individuality."

THE LEGACY OF THE PAST AND THE LATE-TWENTIETH-CENTURY URBAN IMAGINARY

There are clearly limitations to the metaphor of city as body and the city's identity as simply an economic structure. One of those limitations may be the failure to value or even identify the unique forms of cultural and spatial practice which mark urban cultures. However, there are virtues as well to understanding the city whose economy is based on the production or merchandising of goods as a whole, the condition of whose parts depends on economic conditions within the totality of that structure. In part, Booth's recommendations—which, as he points out, were developments already well under way on their own—work because London's economy, which had never been primarily based on primary production, was moving away at that moment even from secondary production. Aves, writing for Booth, calls London "the Mecca of the Anglo-Saxon race," and argues that its economic well-being rests on its status as "Mother City of the Kingdom and the Empire" (*Life* 9: 182) and an "unrivalled national emporium and world market" (*Life* 9: 180). At the same time, he recognizes London as a remarketing and finished goods center rather than a manufactory, since the little manufacturing done in London is departing for the provinces.

Writing of the late twentieth century, David Clark observes that exurbanization is a widespread trend in the developed world, defining it thus: "The most important part of the 'exurbanisation' phase in the spatial evolution of the city is that the population decentralises. . . . [The next stage] is a shift, at the national scale . . . to counterurbanisation" (56). He speculates that this may simply be the next stage in the life cycle of cities. However, this observation ignores that cities are quite different. London exurbanized when it began to become a primary global city, a city whose "manufacturing economy is comparatively small but [which] . . . is the principal supplier of financial and producer services to global markets, a role which it developed as the hub of the British Empire" (Clark 141). This economic development freed London businesses from their ties to the urban core, already tenuous at this time, and enabled their dispersal, as did the movement of trade, as well as production, to the provinces and the northern and western industrial cities.

Exurbanisation and decentralization are often praised by those who believe urban ills are largely produced by size:

> One possibility to realize . . . [the advantages without the disadvantages arising from "gigantism"] is to organize a major metropolis into a constellation city. This is a cluster of self-sufficient cities of 1.5 to 3 million people, [spaced close together in] . . . an attempt to take advantage of today's rapid rail transportation and very efficient expressway system to meet new needs. (Thai-Ker 18)

Thai-Ker cites the example of the British New Towns as justifications for this structure, as well as its success in Singapore.[1] Urban analyst Wilfred Owen also celebrates this vision, asserting that "intercontinental transport and communication have already made us into a world of united cities. The compression of the planet into an integrated world city had its beginnings in the 1950s." He does admit though that the "transport revolution will have to be extended to the vast hinterlands of the globe" before we can truly say we have achieved this (246). He too celebrates decentralization and the New Town model. One wonders, however, what space there is in this vision for analysis of the different roles and developmental patterns of the dependent global cities, as well as the smaller manufacturing centers on which they depend, let alone nonmodernized and rural areas of the world. (Where does, say, Juarez fit into this analysis?)[2] As we focus on the metropolis and the global city, we may be neglecting the dependent manufacturing city and dependent rural areas, still the sine qua nons of global capitalism.

Charles Angotti points out that this model reflects a deeply antiurban theoretical bias, which begins in Anglo-Saxon theories of urban structure upon which the Chicago school was founded. He doesn't mention Booth, beginning instead with Ebenezer Howard, but remarks that these planners "like to use medical metaphors that suggest urban ills can be 'cured' by applying remedial measures (and even surgery, or excision of the 'cancer')" (148).[3] He cites Ernest Burgess of the Chicago school as the first person who, in 1961, "attempted to show how urban settlements grow outward in concentric circles through a process of a succession of land uses and social groups" (155).

Certainly, as we have seen, this emerges quite early on, as Booth's analysis is informed by earlier sanitary mapping. Angotti points out that "all of Britain's New Towns house the equivalent of only 15 per cent of Greater London's population" according to U.S. Deptartment of Labor statistics in 1971 (148), and charges that the valuing of decentralized New Towns over the metropolis "appeals to the most conservative social impulses—a return to small-town living, narrow rural values and the presumed bliss of single-family homeownership. . . . It romanticizes what Karl Marx once called 'the idiocy of rural life.' . . . As politics, it tends to buttress conservative policies ranging from fiscal cutbacks in social services to exclusionary zoning" (148). Pointing out that such theories use Darwinist narratives to posit a natural death cycle for the "outworn" metropolis, which behaves as an organism, Angotti observes that this theory is usually applied to "poor and working class neighborhoods," which then justifies their continued neglect. He connects antiurbanism to "contemporary idealized notions of the neighborhood and community . . . home rule and municipal authority. . . . It usually translates into, or covers up, exclusionary and discriminatory practices. In Europe, it has recently taken the form of rising regionalism and nationalism, in opposition to immigrant populations . . . and to the process of European integration" (150).

It is always a matter of some concern when the solidly right and the moderate left propose the same solutions. Both sides continued in the 1990s to favor decentralization in the management of London. The Right favored a privatized, consumerist approach, positing (much like Booth) that consumption is mostly localized, and therefore that government should reflect that localization. The Left approached decentralization with a language of rights, the championship of local identity and democracy, but still rested the notion of consumer identity on consumption. Against the false exclusionary community of the suburb or new town, Angotti positions the neighborhood as both myth and place. Just why Angotti, however, favors neighborhood government, but not New Town governmental structures, is based on an argument which could have been taken from Booth directly: "Even while production becomes more and more mobile, neighborhood based consumption and reproduction are relatively fixed features. There is evidence that interactions among neighbors are not necessarily affected by a high level of mobility" (Angotti 205).

Robin Hambleton, like Angotti, advocates a very local form of democracy to counteract the problems of a local consumerist approach (255–57).[4] The problem with these formulations, at least in a capitalist system, is that localism always seems to be exalted for the disadvantaged. Neighborhood pride, a sense of local identity, and so on are thought to give poor people a stake (that is, an interest) in civic identity—a version of the mid-nineteenth-century notion of tutelage for citizenship through house pride. One thinks of H. Llewelyn Smith in the Booth reports, rhetorically querying, "Why is there so little local life and sentiment in East London? Why is it hardly possible to conceive an excited throng crying "Well played, Bethnal Green?" (501). Wealthy cosmopolites (literally, "citizens of the world") neither need nor desire such local identity, though they may indeed seek to safeguard their comfort in clearly defined, isolated neighborhoods. These communities are valued less for a warm sense of identity, however, than for their often bland and featureless homogeneity with an ideal of cosmopolitan living. Most people living in them define their communities through professional and consumer relationships that stretch well beyond the geography of neighborhood. The power of pooled consumption among low earning consumers may not compete very equally with the power of wealthier sectors to determine overall civic policy, as Hambleton notes. Hambleton is right to return us to a language of rights rather than simply interests; how, precisely, this is to be made effective remains a question.

There is also a tendency on the left to celebrate the virtues of local attachment and communitarian identity. Although there are certainly good reasons to advocate and protect such identities, they are not necessarily inherently positive or progressive, as Angotti admits. Ethnic nationalism is one such identity, for example. The celebration of local consumption also seems to contradict many of the values in which city life is rooted, at least for the middle classes, especially its multiplicity and diversity, including the freedom to go to other neighborhoods and participate in a wide variety of cultural and consumer activities available precisely because of the size, diversity, and concentration of urban population. As long as neighborhood pride and neighborhood consumption are largely for the disadvantaged, their mixture with a carefully orchestrated democratic system based on local self-determination may be salutary, but is unlikely to significantly compensate for other disadvantages. Fear of the megacity and a turn to a politics—or an aesthetics!—of localism does not seem to be the answer for the Western global metropolis, and in the Western dependent city may often simply be used as an excuse for irresponsibility in government. Nor is the metaphor of the city as gigantic organism growing centrifugally useful in an era of decentered production. We must find new ways to body forth the complex realities of urban structure and urban life.

ENVISIONING THE PERIPHERY

So much for the metropolis. As for the periphery, representation of space still often takes one of two forms. The third-world city is often seen as a cancerous overgrowth or a failed mimicry of cities in the so-called developed world (Mexico City, Rio, Bangkok), whose failed modern transparency is marred with slums and dirt to an even greater extent than the great cities of the developed countries. This is, however, perhaps more a difference of degree than of kind. On the other hand, third-world rural areas are often seen as the still-disease-producing "bad landscape," wild, uncivilized, and ahistorical or—also ahistorical—caught in a moment of the past that becomes both tourist attraction and the target of various forms of economic intervention aimed either at developing the terrain forcibly in a neocapitalist model (the World Bank) or at preserving local custom while still making connection with capitalist markets (various NGOs). These are lands and communities which have not, supposedly, developed and are therefore underdeveloped or developing, but which, once again, are not quite in the present, economically, technologically, and so on.

As for the body of the other, represented by and conflated with the geography of the periphery, there has been a remarkable continuity. As the second epigraph to this chapter makes clear, AIDS has taken the place of cholera in our own global imaginary. Originally perceived as a "filthy" disease, associated with what many denounced as immoral practices, we have gradually come to see it as something less selectively morally punitive. But, as it has become for us less a disease of homosexual men and intravenous drug users; it has also come increasingly to be perceived as a third-world invasion of the West from the diseased landscape and peoples of the underdeveloped world. In part, of course, this is for the very good reason that economic and related infrastructural conditions in much of Africa, India, or Thailand do make for a particularly vulnerable population. But it also has to do with our image of these places as diseased and disease producing, an image which has changed little since nineteenth-century representations of India and Africa.

In any number of current documents on AIDS or Africa, these connections are indispensable. Ambassador Richard C. Holbrooke, addressing the U.S. Senate Committee on Foreign Relations identifies AIDS as one of top three interrelated African problems:

> Mr. Chairman, we have an interest in helping Africa become more peaceful and prosperous. We have an interest in helping Africans resolve their conflicts and rid their societies of horrible diseases like HIV/AIDS. And we have an interest in helping Africa's people build societies based on democracy, liberty and political freedom.
>
> Despite Africa's profound troubles, we cannot simply build a wall around a continent—particularly in world defined by globalization, where borders are even more permeable and the old rules of international politics even less applicable. The mantra "African solutions for African problems" no longer captures either the breadth of the challenge or the effort required for a solution. Africa's problems are the world's problems—and we have to work together globally to find the right solutions. . . .

Perhaps nothing is more illustrative of this point than the scourge of HIV/AIDS and what it's doing to Africa. As recently as a year ago, few would have considered AIDS as part of a discussion of foreign policy (indeed, our idea to hold last January's special Security Council session on AIDS was initially met with some resistance, including from inside the U.S. Mission). But today, few doubt that HIV/AIDS is a top-shelf national security issue, particularly as it relates to Africa. (United States Senate)

There are, of course, real reasons to identify these three things as part of one problem: a serious pandemic's spread is indeed related to war and war-related economic problems, and this pandemic, in turn, threatens political stability. However, it also dwells persistently on the danger of AIDS spreading from Africa when in fact AIDS is already a global pandemic; increasingly, AIDS is identified not as a disease which afflicts Africans, among others, but as an African disease. The continuities between issues that Ambassador Holbrooke identifies as global problems are not here explicitly related to the global economic structure that is certainly at least partially implicated in Africa's health crisis, but to the permeable borders that will allow AIDS to spread (again) beyond Africa and the unstable political situation which will allow refugees and hostility to seep through those porosities as well, destabilizing the surrounding regions.

The identification of AIDS with Africa is powerful and widespread to the point of ideological invisibility. In Anna Forbes's pedagogical AIDS awareness book aimed at young children, the very first thing we learn is: "This book is about a disease called AIDS. AIDS is a very serious (SEER-ee-us) disease. No one knows for sure just how AIDS began. The first people to get sick with AIDS were in central Africa. Most people think it must have started in that part of the world. Now it is all over the world" (5). In a book that is necessarily stripped down to a few basic facts about AIDS in simple language, one wonders how important it is to include, let alone so emphasize that its origins are thought to be African. But this is emphasized over and over in popular coverage.

My point here is not that these authors are somehow wrong or necessarily inaccurate. But the close association of images and themes they draw on suggests a continuity in our cultural imaginary with past ways of perceiving geography which, although not deliberately misleading, were not innocent in their effects and still resonate. A brief *Newsweek* article identifies Africa as the "breeding grounds" of such viruses and manages in a few sentences to relate this to both the theme of weather (here, a metaphor rather than a vehicle for the spread of infection) and the connection of Africa and the Caribbean which was so strongly emphasized in late 1980s coverage of the disease (which particularly demonized Haitians), though this is a 2002 article:

How does a hurricane reach the Caribbean? If you could trace a storm all the way back to its genesis, maybe you'd find a butterfly fanning its wings in West Africa, causing a momentary disturbance that sends stronger currents swirling across the Atlantic. The weather doesn't lend itself to such precise accounting, but plagues sometimes do. Through years of painstaking genetic analysis, researchers have pieced together a convincing account of how the AIDS pandemic emerged. The culpable viruses— HIV-1 and HIV-2—didn't start their careers as human parasites. Both are primate viruses that seem to have gotten lucky in West central Africa. (Cowley 48)

Eileen Stillwaggon, an uncompromising observer of myths about the developing world, argues against the tendency to focus blame disproportionately on factors other than economically related ones for the prevalence of the disease on Africa. As she remarks, most recent work has focused on the immune response of those infected, rather than simply on the pathogen itself. Rates of transmission and the speed at which the disease progresses vary significantly between rich and poor countries, a fact which Stillwaggon convincingly relates to immune system compromise resulting from malnutrition, chronic parasitic illnesses, and other economically based health problems in poor populations. She concludes,

AIDS policy for very poor countries that relies only on behaviour modification is on the wrong track. That approach has been effective in the United States and Europe and has also had some success in Uganda, demonstrating that behaviour modification is an important element of prevention. But transmission depends on much more than sexual contact, as the low heterosexual transmission rates in rich countries indicate. (22)

Yet, as Stillwaggon remarks, this differential is still often ascribed purely to a behavioral model:

The assumption that the prevalence of HIV can be explained by rates of sexual activity is not something that was left behind in the 1980s or that appears only in the popular press. In the AIDS Update 1999 published by the United Nations Population Fund, the argument is made quite explicitly. 'The problem is promiscuity, and underscores the primacy of cultural factors,' the report proclaims on page six in a special box on the subject. . . . An implicit assumption or explicit assertion of higher rates of sexual partner change in Africa appears in numerous works. (22)

In short, in the works Stillwaggon criticizes here, we once again have the bad landscape (with its bad fauna) and the bad behavior of its inhabitants—shades of India's pestilential alluvial soil and incorrigible religious pilgrims. Yet, even

though Stillwaggon is critical of these statements, she (unconsciously? ironically?) draws on the metaphorical entailments of nineteenth-century notions of
intrinsic disease, and on twentieth-century associations of Africa and Africans
with diseased earth, in her title: "HIV/AIDS in Africa: Fertile Terrain."

PERIPHERAL DISEASE AND THE METROPOLITAN BODY

I have quoted here at length from an eclectic selection of texts to make a
point: in discourses aimed at our children, a popular readership, the Senate,
and even epidemiological specialists, some vestige of the Victorian association
of the economic periphery with stagnated development, premodern space, and
the diseased Other casts its long shadow over our perceptions of geography.
Of course, the association with AIDS and Africa and its peculiar history has
been addressed by many scholars, and so my point here is hardly a new one.
But I wished here to point to the persistence of two strands in the figuration
of the peripheral landscape from the Victorian period: first, as both diseased
and caught in static past time, and second, as a threat, through disease and disorder, to the modern metropole. The economic bases of a population's vulner-
abilty are still often ascribed to landscape and ethnic behavioral peculiarites in
preference to infrastructural problems, whereas in the developed world, infrastructure (after initial resistance) is now widely though not universally understood to be paramount. This, of course, is primarily a problem of cost. But it
is also a problem of imagination, a world in which AIDS is not just a disease
that happens to be in Africa, but is quintessentially an African disease, something that, in the popular imaginary of the West, belongs in Africa.

Where it does not belong, in this narrative, is in the West. In the early
1980s, this theme was very apparent in the coverage. A typical example from
the *Chicago Tribune* reads, "According to some prevalent theories, AIDS is
thought to have originated in Central Africa, probably Zaire. Haitians and
Frenchmen working there carried the disease back to Haiti and Paris. From
Haiti it spread to New York and Miami and then on to San Francisco and Los
Angeles" (Kotulak 11). These narratives often tend to elide the spread from,
say, the United States to Latin America, although often these facts are
acknowledged in the details of the same document. Nor has this attitude significantly changed. In 1993, Dr. Upton stated in the Irish Parliament,

> Problems such as environmental degradation, ethnic conflicts, population
> growth, AIDS and other diseases, will not be limited or mainly centred in
> underdeveloped countries. They are global problems; they develop in one
> place and then spread to developed countries. For example, AIDS is believed
> to have originated in Africa, although some microbiologists and medical

people might put forward arguments about that. It is now a major problem in western society. This is clearly related to the fact that its development in Africa was totally without control for a long time. Western society remained indifferent to the problems of Africa and it is now experiencing its own terrible problems as a result.

Here, the problems of Africa are blamed on Western neglect, but they are seen as indeed African problems, and the spread of disease to the developed world, after developing "in one place" which is clearly not anywhere in the developed world. That AIDS in Africa developed "totally without control," overlooking any of the local efforts which have been made to control it or the differences between African nations, is taken for granted. Further, this uncontrolled development is read as prior to AIDS having become a problem in Western countries, when of course its presence as a pandemic in several Western countries was a serious problem before the African problem was even diagnosed.

Turning to a different example, the recent hysteria over West Nile virus (WNV) in the United States, the name's suggestiveness of African origins has confused many. The website of a U.S. pediatric clinic explains, "West Nile Virus, normally found in Africa and Asia, spread to New York City in 1999. This year it has spread to many other areas of the country" (Oconee Pediatrics). Yet the Center for Disease Control (CDC) identifies the strain afflicting North America as more closely aligned with Middle Eastern ones as well as with St. Louis encephalitis, endemic to the Americas for quite some time before the arrival of the West Nile variant: "West Nile virus has been commonly found in humans and birds and other vertebrates in Africa, Eastern Europe, West Asia, and the Middle East. . . . It is not known from where the U.S. virus originated, but it is most closely related genetically to strains found in the Middle East." It has also been in western Europe since at least the 1960s, but by identifying the virus's origins with Africa, Asia, and sometimes the Middle East, most sources of public information imply that it came to the United States directly from these places, which is not yet known. In fact, North Carolina's Division of Environmental Health website explicitly and incorrectly states that "West Nile Virus, *previously restricted to Africa, West Asia and the Middle East,* has recently been found in New York" (emphasis added).

Once again, it is entirely possible that West Nile did arrive, by chance, from Africa, and probable that it happened to enter through New York, as we are fairly sure AIDS did; New York is a major point of entry into the United States. But what is interesting is the insistence on this model of developing to developed world transmission, from the rural third world to the urban first. It is entirely possible that WNV entered through New Jersey or Maryland. It is quite possible that the first AIDS victim in Argentina caught the virus from a New Yorker, or in New York, or for that matter, from a small-town-U.S.

Midwesterner. But these are not readily imagined or oft repeated narratives. Plagues come from Africa, and invade the great Western cities—the vectors of the otherwise healthy developed world—and thence travel both to the heartland and the far corners of the globe. The great body of the teeming city is the site of vulnerability to foreign diseases; those diseases originate, epizootically, from the jungles of the animalized third world. The rotten core of the overgrown city is the racialized fifth column through which diseases of the periphery enter and conquer the metropole. Like Victorians who could not see the cholera marching north or east—only west—what we perceive is shaped by our expectations, racial and spatial.

In *Bruno and Sylvie Concluded*, Lewis Carroll wrote of mapmakers whose desire to be precise (and to improve on British mapmakers from whom they learned their craft) defeated their project: having made a map at a 1-to-1 ratio, they were unable to open it, for fear of covering the entire country. In his absurd story, this causes no problems, for they simply "use the country itself, as its own map, and I assure you it does nearly as well." In this afterword, I have attempted to very briefly indicate some of the continuities in the perception of space and geography which enable us to trace the past in the present—indeed, which lead us to ask the questions I have explored here of the past in the first place. The nineteenth-century moment of medical mapping and the cholera epidemics that gave the project its urgent impetus have been epistemologically foundational for our views of space and health, of the metropole and the margin. Maps, visual and verbal, transform as well as reflect. The ways of seeing learned from the early years of disease mapping has left on the land itself the most durable of inscriptions. In this way the terrain comes to be produced by that which purports merely to represent it: the land itself indeed becomes its own map.

NOTES

PREFACE

1. I have limited the scope of the domestic end of this project to England, both because of its importance in metropolitan representation and because the trajectory of Scottish and Irish sanitary projects differed in their administrative and representational development, and a detailed study of the comparisons are beyond the scope of a single study. In dealing with imperial representations of a disease perceived to be "colonial" in nature, it is essential, however, to always maintain awareness of the mutually constitutive roles of "center" and "periphery"; it is to this end that the study juxtaposes representations in London and in India.

CHAPTER 1. MAPPING AND SOCIAL SPACE IN NINETEENTH-CENTURY ENGLAND

1. As Thomas Richards has discussed at length in *The Imperial Archive.*

2. Physical space in the nineteenth century has been understood largely in Euclidean terms and is therefore susceptible of measurement seeking to homogenize it.

3. I am following here the tradition of Anglo-American urbanists in my distinction between the terms "place" and "space." Translations of de Certeau have used these terms in an inverse relation to this tradition, which has created a certain amount of confusion. Given the way we use these terms in English, it seems to make more sense to use them in the way detailed above.

4. Interestingly, Golledge notes, cognitive uses of such remembered or internalized formal maps seem to be no more accurate spatially than more directly experiential organizations of space.

5. Massey observes that

the identities of places are inevitably unfixed . . . in part because the social relations out of which they are constructed are themselves by their very nature dynamic and changing . . . [and] the past was not more static than the present. Places cannot 'really' be characterized by the recourse to some essential, internalized moment . . . [seeking] the identity of a place by laying claim to some particular moment/location in time-space when the definition of the area and the social relations dominant within it were to the advantage of that particular claimant group. (169)

Massey notes that this is typical of nationalistic spatial claims.

6. Map companies routinely sold embroidery patterns, where the maps were printed on fabric; in the 1790s, Bowles and Carvers offered twenty such patterns ranging from the Northern Hemisphere to "Twenty Miles Round Oxford" (Tyner 6). Cartographic production was unprecedented and quite large in this period, both independently and as a result of the ordinance survey's activities.

7. Thrower notes that a fifty-sheet hand atlas, published in 1817–22, and inexpensive wall maps made cartographic representations "available to large numbers of students and the general public. The use of globes, maps and atlases also became important school subjects for both girls and boys at this time" (*Maps and Civilization* 125). Obviously, the general public here is at least middle class. Still, this is a significant change in the public conception of the world. At the lower end of the market, between 1830 and 1843, the Society for the Diffusion of Useful Knowledge (SDUK) was publishing a series of maps of principal cities of the world for their audience (Thrower, *Maps and Civilization* 140). SDUK publications were usually aimed at literate but not highly educated artisans with an interest in self-improvement, in other words, the relatively comfortable working class.

8. By 1853, for example, the National Society for Promoting Education of the Poor produced several publications such as the twenty-eight-page *Geography of Asia with a Map* in 16o size. This pamphlet and others like it included many facts and a useful foldout map for 1s 6d per dozen. The text assumes familiarity with maps and ready access to maps and globes on the part of its audience, though it doesn't presuppose very sophisticated map use. For example, it carefully explains scale so that readers looking at a similar map of Britain or Europe will understand the difference in size between areas represented on similar sized paper. Travel guides, such as Chez Baily Frere's pocket-sized *Londres et Ses Environs* (1862), a volume comprised of six "rambles through London" originally printed in the *Cornhill*, contained a foldout map of London with itineraries picked out in a single color, for a shilling. There were several English editions, and it was translated into a number of foreign languages. By the late 1860s, inexpensive schoolbooks for children were rife with maps. Miss Corner's *The History of England from the Earliest Period to the Present Time Adapted to Youth, Schools and their Families* was under two shillings, and that is how most volumes, all liberally provided with maps and advertised in the same series, were priced. The 1870 edition of Miss Corner's volume that I examined was in its 83rd thousandth printing. These are a few examples out of countless possibilities. In short, maps were widely cognitively available as a mode of spatial perception by the mid-nineteenth century. And, of course, map use created a new category of cognitive difference between the map literate and illiterate, linked to class difference, and moving ever farther down the social scale as the century advanced.

9. Londoners were eager to place themselves in their city and to master its codes, including an elaborate code of social hierarchies by address. It is no accident that several midcentury magazines aiming themselves at the upwardly mobile lower middle class were named after upscale neighborhoods, such as *Belgravia*, a journal conducted by M. E. Braddon. Londoners not only understood themselves as situated within London, but as defined through the city and its narratives.

10. Again, mapmaking was widely taught. William Hughes's preface to the second edition of his textbook mentions that it has been translated into Urdu and is in use in the Civil Engineering College in India. J. Bailey Denton, in a paper addressed to town surveyors and cartographers, remarks, "It is quite unnecessary in these days when land drainage and town sewerage are objects of general consideration to dwell upon the first necessity of a knowledge of altitudes when dealing with water" (5).

11. The autographic technique involved printing from the plate onto a surface, and then using that surface to make the final print. This obviated the need to create the image on the plate in reverse, thus enabling less skilled workmen to create the plates, and also made it easier to create overlays, and after 1850, to print colors (Robinson *Early Thematic Mapping* 188–89). See Robinson for a more detailed discussion of mapmaking techniques.

12. In addition, Petermann's 1852 map used variable shading to show density of cholera victims. Furthermore, different kinds of maps had been used to convey medical information. Although most are flat maps, Michaelis's 1843 map uses contours to connect incidence of cretinism to elevation and Acland's 1855 cholera map of Oxford also uses contours to show elevation.

13. Delaporte quotes French authorities' response to the cholera epidemic of 1832. In order to research their report,

> A map of Paris was first cut up into forty-eight quartiers, each of which was copied onto a separate sheet of paper to form a new map of individual neighborhoods, so that it became possible to see at a glance the widely varying size of the neighborhoods, their sometimes bizarre shapes, and the way in which these various sections of the capital were situated. (Benoiston de Chateauneuf, *Rapport sur le Marché et les effets de cholera-morbus dans Paris* [1834] in Delaporte 73–74)

14. E. W. Gilbert outlines the following as the major English cholera maps, and in so doing gives some idea of the range of techniques already in use by the first half of the century: Robert Baker's 1833 map of Leeds, wherein affected areas were colored red in flat tones; W. P. Ormerod's 1848 sanitary condition map of Oxford, showing cholera and fever districts for 1832 (marked by a dot and cross respectively), with faintly shaded areas to show spaces prone to "disease generally"; Thomas Shapter's 1849 dot map of Exeter, also showing the cholera epidemic of 1832; distinguished cartographer Augustus Petermann, when he established himself in London, inaugurated his work in England with a cholera map of the whole British Isles, also for the 1832 epidemic; John Snow's famous 1855 dot map showed deaths in the area surrounding the Broad Street pump (and, though Gilbert doesn't mention it explicitly, clearly his

other map of 1855 showing the distribution of cholera in relation to two water companies belongs on this list); and finally Henry Wentworth Acland's cholera maps of Oxford (1856), showing all three epidemics to that date, the contours of the city at intervals of five feet, and several other factors.

Of course, there were many other disease maps which were published abroad, yet were well known and influential in Britain. The early spot maps of yellow fever in the United States which Stevenson describes had probably been seen by many medical writers of the period. Although they would have had little or no impact on geographer-cartographers such as Petermann, many of the important medical maps and most of the earliest ones were created not by cartographers but by medics mapping disease onto inexpensive existing maps or drawings from such maps. Still, those maps in turn influenced cartographers, who created much more sophisticated representations. (Medics tended to map particular incidences for specific purposes, whereas professionals like Berghaus and Petermann created larger, more overarching maps and series including multiple variables.)

Jarcho identifies five cholera maps produced from 1820 to 1831 which focus on India or India and Asia. ("Yellow Fever"). However, many more were produced which include Europe and Africa and slightly later world maps were frequently used (Stevenson 228). Most concentrate on showing lines of spread, and some include dates of onset and names of locations. (Lines of spread were still popular in 1832; Jarcho cites twenty-two cholera maps produced in 1832 alone, most of which show lines of spread.)

In Germany, Heinrich Berghaus, who trained Petermann, produced the immediately internationally popular *Physikalisher Atlas* in installments from 1845 to 1848, with two subsequent revised editions. In addition to several other large categories, the atlas included an anthropographic section with four subsections: the first included race, nutrition, population, birth and death rates, stature, and physical strength; the second was a geographic distribution of human diseases, including insets on cholera, mental disease, goiter, onset of puberty and senescence, and diseases characteristic of North America and the West Indies; the third showed types of clothing; and the fourth showed occupation, religion and government (Jarcho, "The Contributions" 413–14). As Jarcho notes, this is an important innovation, since it is the first medical map which shows both endemic and epidemic disease (previous maps tend to focus on epidemic disease) and the first medical maps to be in an atlas (414).

We might also note that within this Borgesian list of topics, disease itself, as well as other areas we would consider medical, has a very important place. The anthropographic section itself is one of only eight in the atlas (the others include meteorology/climatology, hydrography, geology, telluric magnetism, botanical geography, zoological geography, and ethnography (Jarcho, "The Contributions" 413).

The first thematic maps of language, religion, race and so forth gave way to population maps (including Petermann's famous population map of Britain) and by the 1850s included sophisticated economic maps (again Petermann's great exhibition maps of 1851 come to mind).

15. Many excellent studies following Margaret Pelling's magisterial *Cholera, Fever and English Medicine* have detailed the multifaceted debate between the contagionists and anticontagionists, two large artificial categories created largely by political pres-

sures to take a firm stand on the issue of whether or not cholera was contagious (a category that could include "infectious") in order to approve or disapprove economically problematic quarantines on goods and travelers. In fact, most medics held theories which are not so easily categorized. Those include contingent contagionist theories (that under some circumstances a noncontagious disorder could become contagious) and theories of atmospheric predisposition as well as the more popularly known miasmatic theories. Chadwick is largely associated with the latter, and medics often aligned themselves with miasmatic theories as acceptable popular substitutes for professional theories too complex to communicate easily to the public. This topic is too large to address at length here, but the popular and political division of these complex ideas into these two simple categories continues to inform the public's understanding of cholera and medics' responses to it for much of the century.

16. Poovey provides an excellent history of the concept of a fact as a unit of knowledge separable from theoretical knowledge through the seventeenth and eighteenth centuries, and the invention of this concept in response to the need to create a knowledge separable from politics. She also demonstrates that this concept of the fact was always under fire from those who considered such knowledge to be inseparable from theories. Here, however, we will be concerned with the practical history of medical knowledge widely considered to be factual, because numerable and susceptible of representation in charts and cartograms, a business largely carried on without a great deal of reference to what had become by the midnineteenth century a largely academic and philosophical debate about the relationship of facts to induction.

CHAPTER 2. VISIBLE AT A GLANCE:
ENGLISH SANITARY AND MEDICAL MAPS

1. I have translated Foucault's term *savoirs* in this way instead of simply using "knowledges" in order to underscore that these are active techniques of knowing that imply the ability to change the object of knowledge, rather than simply bodies of information.

2. I am using Frank Mort's term "medics" to indicate the broad body of medical practitioners in this period who considered themselves professionals (that is, not just those titled "doctors," but surgeons, apothecaries, and later in the period surgeon-apothecaries and general practitioners). The term "sanitarians" generally refers to those who espoused sanitary theories—that is, that dirt and the overcrowding that created it were responsible for epidemic disease. This included many medics, but also laymen such as Edwin Chadwick.

3. For an excellent example, see Thomas C. E. Hawksley, *Replies to the Queries issued by Her Majesty's Commissioners for inquiring into the present State of Large Towns &c., with additional observations in answer to the further inquiries of J. R. Martin*, which includes several maps, plans, and diagrams, showing locations of individual homes in some areas with privies, and so on.

4. The description in the woodcut explanations reads, "Dipping Steps Under the Battery. These steps are situated under the portion of the town wall so termed. The

stream is one of the mill leats that flow through the lower part of the city. The whole scene is now much changed, the dipping steps are bricked up on each side, and a perpendicular wall rises from the leat; the houses on the town wall have been removed, by which means a great improvement has been effected, air and light being thus admitted into two of the principal and densely occupied streets of the south-western quarter" (7). Note the emphasis on change and progress.

5. All citations of Acland in this chapter are from the *Memoir,* unless otherwise indicated.

6. In fact, Ormerod and Acland were old friends and corresponded regularly for many years.

7. He also indicates by a broken brown line drawn into the watercourses (colored blue) where rivers are contaminated with sewage, and with a brown triangle where sewage is entering the watercourse. Buildings are picked out in beige. Undrained districts are shaded in green. The map also includes large brown dots to show areas described by Ormerod, and brown circles to show areas described by Ormerod which have been remedied, as well as showing areas defined as problematic by other writers. (Acland here follows the tradition of using a color scheme that is partly representative—for example, blue water—and partly conventional—for example, illness is dark.)

8. Spot maps have a tendency to visually convey the impression of a static population overtaken by disease, a combination of their visual characteristics and their sanitarian history. Maps with lines of spread show a human practice of space-time over a geographic field, thus focusing on human agency and, of course, almost always implying contagion or, as we have come to understand later, at least a disease whose reservoir is at lest partially in human flesh. Date spot maps can be used for either, both, or neither, though their mapping of time onto space implies an active agency rather than an "epidemic constitution" of the earth; this can be human or another living vector or, as it was so often in Victorian times, meteorological activity.

9. For example, Matthew Arnold suggests that "culture indefatigably tries, not to make what each raw person may like, the rule by which he fashions himself; but to draw ever nearer to a sense of what is indeed beautiful, graceful, and becoming, and to get the raw person to like that" (11).

CHAPTER 3. INVISIBLE TO THE NAKED EYE: JOHN SNOW

1. Brody et al.

2. Narrative also continued its role of appealing to the emotions. As it was increasingly relegated to the use of recounting individual and even aberrant stories, it also made the pathetic appeal for identification with a sufferer that mobilized consent for the allocation of resources. But this function was increasingly separated from scientific and medical writing over the course of the century and reserved for more popular venues.

3. Furthermore, Marcus notes, such manifestations were associated with the rental house and the transience of its inmates, with all the threats to middle-class norms of domesticity that implied, threats associated with unsanitary conditions and disease: "Ghosts also conferred on middle-class houses the contagion and illness that urban investigators like Chadwick had associated with the housing of the poor" (125).

4. See P. Gilbert, "'Scarcely To Be Described,'" for a fuller discussion.

5. See, for example, his letter in the *Edinburgh Medical Journal*. Snow also disputes the accuracy of findings of the General Board in the 1857 *British Medical Journal*.

6. Farr is amusingly exasperated with those who use statistics fallaciously. He refutes critics of the waterborne theory, noting that some argue that many houses supplied with East London water show no cases of cholera, but "Eels, as we have seen, were found in the water of a certain number of houses in East London. To argue that in . . . other houses no eels were found, and that therefore the company never distributed eels in the district, would be absurd" (*Report on the Cholera* xxv).

7. He also refers to problems caused by incorrect maps and other information about communication between water company lines and certain reservoirs: "Neither Wyld's map nor Stanford's map shows the underground iron pipe; hence the omission of its notice in the Weekly Return of July 28th, which gave the company a legitimate ground of complaint and a defence, until the other facts were discovered" (*Report on the Cholera* 100).

CHAPTER 4. A TALE OF TWO PARISHES: PLACE AND NARRATIVE IN THE LONDON CHOLERA EPIDEMIC OF 1854

1. For our purposes here, it is necessary to remind ourselves of the distinction between physical spaces—that is, areas of the city, defined topographically, which are filled with a variety of features, geographical, built, lived, and so on—and what Lefebvre calls "perceived social spaces," and I will here, following a tradition in urban geographical scholarship, call "places," which are apprehended through a name, understood symbolically, and incorporate political, cultural, social, and mythical elements.

2. Place becomes one narrative, one lens—a most powerful one—through which the city and the nation it represents can be understood. Such a narrative can be powerful enough to elide the narratives of the resident who, after all, only lives there—especially residents whose economic and social position place them in a subject position, a site, in which participation as a subject of the national narrative in which their location is mythically implicated is limited.

3. Benedict Anderson has remarked that the place of the imagined community, like its language, is both historically determined and empty of history. In the same way that the nation imagines a shared history, and yet the nation as a concept exists outside of historical time, the imagined place is both historically specific and eternal. Hence, although projects to tear down the Rookery may be imagined, St. Giles (per se) as other than St. James's dark twin could not be conceived. (It is telling that long

after the particular slum known as "the Rookery" was pulled down, the surrounding slums continued to be called by that name.) St. Giles as a historical space is amenable to urban renewal projects such as Shaftesbury's; as a mythic place, it is not. In fact, today St. Giles as a place has ceased to exist. The church remains and a few signs testify to its presence and to the former identity of the district, but St. Giles as a community has vanished into Bloomsbury and Holborn. Thoroughly absorbed and rehabilitated, it no longer has a reason to be, Soho having eclipsed it as a symbolically rich district. Were it not immortalized in the "Bells" song, the entire idea of St. Giles might well be lost entirely. St. James's is obviously in no such danger.

4. Again, this is a most uneven development. Realist fiction is full of predetermined bodies marked by phrenology and other hereditary and humoral markers. We are talking about a general trend, not a precise and clearly marked paradigm shift.

5. In *Selling Spaces,* Kearns and Philo remark, "Central to the activities subsumed under the heading of selling places is often a conscious and deliberate manipulation of culture in an effort to enhance the appeal and interest of places. . . . In part this . . . depends upon promoting traditions, lifestyles and arts that are supposed to be locally rooted" (3). Kearns and Philo are discussing the late-twentieth-century practice of marketing places to tourists and investors, but there are some interesting parallels in the nascent understanding of London as a tourist attraction—an attraction precisely based on its status as the omphalos of Empire—consolidated in the period preceding the 1851 Exhibition.

6. Today's marketers take advantage of ways of perceiving places that have been in existence for some time. In current marketing practice, Kearns and Philo observe, "An additional key ingredient . . . is that of history. . . . It is evident that the culture of a place, however this might be understood, is intimately bound up with the history of that place and with the histories . . . of the peoples who have ended up living in that place" (4). Unfortunately, however, "the cultural and historical appropriations of the bourgeoisie [and the marketers] frequently do appear untenable when put alongside the alternative cultural and historical appropriations made by the 'other peoples' of the city," meaning the nonmajority dwellers (27). Certainly this is operative in the case of St. James's, whose citizenry lodged in the relatively poor area of Broad Street had a very different perception of their home parish than implied to most metropolitan residents and consumers of the metropolis by courtly St. James's.

7. See also "Seven Dials" and "The Pawnbroker's Shop" among the *Sketches,* as well as several mentions in *Household Words.*

8. See especially Keating's *The Working Classes in Victorian Fiction* and the Introduction to *Into Unknown England.* Nancy Aycock Metz extends this analysis to argue that such representations overlap with and are shaped increasingly by narrative techniques associated with sensational fiction in the 1860s.

9. On choleraphobia and its results, see the extensive literature on cholera in the nineteenth century, especially Durey and Morris for England, Rosenberg for the United States, Delaporte and Kudlick for France, and Evans for Germany.

10. It is interesting to note that the mythic narrative of urban space was much more resistant than the apparently more culturally basic mythic narrative of sanitari-

anism. However, the sanitary narrative was newer, contained the seeds of its own destruction, and was under assault from more directions. It is also possible that, as places are obviously mythologized unevenly, St. James's and St. Giles were so resistant to rereading because of the long histories which had given the myths weight. Just as public places are more important in reading place than private ones, and older structures generally more crucial to the inflexibility of place identity than newly built ones, it may be possible that natural features are more easily mythologized than built ones. Ultimately, modernity is represented by the abstraction and therefore malleability of space—the modern, Bauhaus-inspired office block may be less susceptible of mythic narration than the brooding Gothic cathedral not only because it is newer, or less "romantic" in appearance, but because its very nature fundamentally indicates the malleability of space—its potential to be restructured at a moment's notice—which is hostile to mythic narrative's dependence on permanence. Thus, St. Giles's was destroyed as an imagined entity by the Oxford New Cut and the redistribution of parish boundaries, despite the persistence of the slum (the Rookery) which had always defined it and the church (still in place today) which was the parish's namesake. Even by the time Dickens wrote of the Rookery as Tom All Alone's in *Bleak House,* it could only be described as located in "part of Holborn."

CHAPTER 5. MEDICAL MAPPING, THE THAMES,
AND THE BODY IN DICKENS'S *OUR MUTUAL FRIEND*

1. It is important to remember that feces' categorization and value fluctuated with various reclamation programs through the midcentury. Still, fecal material within the city was generally viewed with disgust.

2. In short, models of illness fluctuated in grossly the same terms as models of economic responsibility: between an individual as a closed system responsible for itself and a communitarian notion of a porous body vulnerable to outside influences often beyond its control.

3. A word is in order here about the use of the term "liberal," which may surprise readers steeped in Dickens's rejection of classical liberal economics and his obvious insistence on social connection and responsibility in many of his works. There were many kinds of liberals, of course, in mid-Victorian society, and Dickens is more a later Millsian than Smithian liberal, emphasizing social responsibility while retaining a largely Kantian notion of a core individual self. But most importantly, Dickens is drawing on an iconographic, literary, and medical tradition of the Enlightenment middle-class body (and subject) which emphasizes individualism and separation, a tradition of representation which radically undermines a notion of connected society and, indeed, positions it as a threat.

4. John Kucich has traced this dichotomy in several of Dickens's novels. Reading the relationship as essentially one between that of the formlessness implicit in death and the conservative impulse toward life, following Bataille, he sees the novels as staging death, through loss, deaths, overspending, and the like, in order ultimately

to recuperate order and restraint. Kucich also remarks the tendency of Dickens's heroes to achieve integration through some scene of disintegration, whether of violence or of expenditure (108). Kucich's fine reading concentrates on a psychoanalytic vision of the self, but his key opposition between excess and restraint, between disintegration and self-control, is one I will explore here in terms of the relation of the individual's body to the social body and the city.

5. Many scholars have discussed the contents of the dustheaps, and whether we are to take them as containing feces or not. Setting aside the historical question of their likely contents, we should look at the literary question of their representation. In the light of that question, there seems to be little doubt that the dustheaps are waste and represent, at least allegorically, human waste. Critics have noted the anality of *Our Mutual Friend* (see especially Steig and Gallagher) and the fecal equation with filthy lucre. I would like to suggest that both greed and the abjected material of the body represent its dependence on others and lack of closure, its susceptibility to the mass humanity of barbarism/anarchy, rather than the clean liberal individualism and bodily closure of civilization/culture.

6. Hopkins and Read place her death in Henley on Thames and the lock in Hurley. However, much textual evidence suggests that this is incorrect. First, Betty walks to the border but not beyond it, and Henley is a full mile beyond the border. Second, the village is quite small, as is Hurley, not a fair sized town like Henley. It is likely that Betty dies near Hurley. Further, Betty walks part of a night and a full, long day from the lock. Given that she is lost part of the time, she still walks a good eighteen to twenty hours, at least twelve or so of which are in one direction. Hurley and Henley are only approximately five miles apart as the river runs. Betty has walked much further than that. So regardless of whether she dies at Hurley or Henley, the lock cannot be at Hurley. Between the time Betty passes the lock and the time she dies, she notices water meadows, which suggest the marshy area near Windsor, anywhere between Staines and Slough, though it might also be further up, closer to her final destination.

Furthermore, Eugene sculls by the lock in the late afternoon, and puts up at an inn substantially upriver from there in the evening, to continue on at 6 a.m.; it is unlikely he would stop for the night if he were very close to his destination. When Bradley leaves the lock to follow Eugene, he does not return for approximately thirty-three to thirty-eight hours (637). Some of this time is spent shadowing Eugene, of course, having already caught up with him. But he says he returns immediately, without rest, to the lock, having seen Eugene, and we know Eugene sees Lizzie in the evening after work. Still, having left again to go back to Eugene between three and five o'clock or so in the morning (637), it takes a full day again to catch up with Eugene, as the night Headstone assaults Eugene shortly after full darkness (probably around midnight) is two nights after his first arrival. It takes him that night and the following day and night to return; he arrives between 2:00 and 3:00 a.m. (703). Headstone says he has not rested; even allowing for time hiding on the road, he has left the village before news of Lizzie's finding Eugene reached him. It is reasonable, then to assume that the lock is at least twelve to sixteen hours downriver from Hurley or Henley on foot, at a conservative estimate, twenty-five miles, assuming that Betty was lost and slow and Bradley was not travelling a direct route. It seems likely that Riderhood's lock is near Windsor, past

Staines, as he says, twenty to twenty-five miles "and odd" from London, from near Hyde Park (551). That would place him near Windsor, following the road (and considerably further east—near Sunbury—if he is following the river, but then he wouldn't be west of Staines, which seems unlikely). It is most definitely not as far as Henley, over fifty miles from London. He is, in short, substantially past the area where the river was being polluted. If in the early 1850s Thames Ditton was safe and clean, by the mid-1860s, with urban growth along the river, Dickens may have wanted to go further upstream. The multiple references to place I have cited here suggest something of the precision with which setting is mapped in the novel, and point to the importance that identifying the correct location has in tracking the novel's construction of meaning.

7. The women of the novel, with the exception of Bella and Mrs. Lammle, are largely innocent of the sins for which the men must be purified. Although, as Helena Michie, among others, has pointed out, women suffer for the sins of others in this novel, women do not have power to become protagonists in healing the social body, though they can midwife the healing of male bodies. Nor are they marked by class as are the men; Lizzie and Betty are essentially bourgeois women in working-class clothing. The gender and class politics of the novel's exhortation to self-development are fascinating. Only middle-class men can develop this closure; working-class men who attempt to develop middle-class closure, such as Headstone and Jesse Hexam, are treated as upstarts.

8. Alan Woodcourt returns to Esther having saved his fellow passengers in a shipwreck. One might think also of Kingsley's *Water Babies* as an example of the most basic operation of the archetype of the intiatory sea voyage, and, in the midcentury, its sanitary entailments.

9. This also includes a project of eliminating barbaric others from the metropolitan center by making them like the self. This requires that the British be less preoccupied with others abroad, who are geographically and personally resistant to such transformation. (Jo cannot be civilized because the Mrs. Jellybys of the world are preoccupied with Borrioboola-Gha, in which the king, much like Mr. Wilfer's cheap and nasty African king, is constitutionally unable to appreciate the British plan for free trade, outside of selling everyone into slavery for rum.) Increasingly, the water and ships come to represent the barbarism of an England in touch with the outside world, with empire, with the other.

CHAPTER 6. INDIA IN THE 1830s:
MAPPING FROM THE PROFESSIONAL PERIPHERY

1. See, for example, David Arnold's analysis of the association of effeminacy with the tropics, especially as applied to Bengal *(The Problem of Nature)*.

2. For example, the zamindari system of land ownership engineered by the British encouraged what Klein calls a "crazy quilt of irrigation" systems which, he argues, caused the degradation of natural waterways in Bengal and their ability to cleanse themselves ("Imperialism" 512).

3. Farr developed this same argument, with much of the same text, in his *Report on the Mortality of Cholera in England 1848–1849*, published in 1852.

4. Interestingly, it also formulated something very like WHO's current call for a global right to healthy environment: "The Conference 'demands for every man pure and abundant air, pure water, and a pure soil' . . . these elements should constitute the 'permanent privilege of populations'" (lxxxix).

5. Susan Gole flatly states that she has not been able to find "any maps of India made before the advent of the Europeans. Geographical treatises there were, both in India and the Middle East. But the idea of a pictorial representation was either absent, or very rudimentary among the Arab geographers" (preface, no page number). In his foreword to Gole's book, Irfan Habib politely demurs, noting that two sets of documents in Persian do exist, the first made by Hamdullah Mustaufi in 1329–40, and the second by Sadiq Isfahini in 1647, which are recognizable maps by Western standards, with legends and so on. Still, he concedes that "modern maps of India trace back their pedigree entirely to European map-making of the sixteenth century. The traditions of map-making in India and the eastern countries that existed earlier have had no effect on modern cartography" (foreword, no page number).

However, there was, in fact, a lively cartographic tradition in India when Europeans arrived. The Persian tradition, which, again, created documents easily recognizable to Westerners as maps, was quite active. Geographic writings were combined with historical writings and gave Europeans much useful information that went into the earliest maps. Thomas Maurice attributes the invention of geography to India and refers extensively to textual descriptions of geography by both Roman and Indian authors. Much of his material is taken from *Ayeen Akbar (The Mirror of Akbar)* including a non-Western map he reproduces as a foldout in volume 1. Much indigenous cartography in the Hindu and Buddhist traditions seems to have been organized around a religious conception of space; D. C. Sircar refers to maps dating back to the eleventh century which, much like European maps of the same period, illustrated a conception of the world founded on a contemporary cosmology, showing a world based on "seven concentric islands, each one of them encircled by a sea" (329). He also refers to Indian-produced charts of the Indian ocean which may have been better for purposes of navigation than European charts of the Mediterranean in the thirteenth through fifteenth centuries. In 1808, British orientalist F. Wilford cautioned, "The Hindus have no name, either for geography or geometry, but we are not to infer thence, that they have entirely neglected those two sciences" (267). He went on to observe,

> Besides geographical tracts, the Hindus have also maps of the world, both according to the system of the Paur'an'ics, and of the astronomers: the latter are very common. They also have maps of India, and of particular districts. . . . The best map . . . was one of the kingdom of Napa'l. . . . The roads were represented by a red line, and the rivers with a blue one. The various ranges were very distinct . . . it wanted but a *scale*. The valley . . . was accurately delineated: but toward the borders of the map, everything was crowed [*sic*], and in confusion. (271)

But Wilford also points out that the Indian maps prefer gorgeous imagery to truth and comments, "Geographical truth is sacrificed to a symmetrical arrangement of countries, mountains, lakes and rivers, with which they are highly delighted" (272). He writes further, "There are two geographical systems among the Hindus . . . the first . . . in which the Earth is considered as a convex surface gradually sloping toward the borders, and surrounded by the ocean" (274). The other organizes the representation of the earth through metaphorical or religious models—of the body or the lotus—with Mount Meru in the middle. But Wilford also observes that the Indians' history is really all myth and that the geography, especially of the second kind, is totally subordinated to those demands. Apparently he also believes there is an aesthetic element which overrides geographical truth in these representations.

The article, however, is a remarkable engagement with the native tradition, despite its condescension. Wilford, instead of dismissing the geography depicted in the maps out of hand, does a careful analysis which tries to transliterate, as it were, the identity of the landmarks and locations depicted in the most popular circular map of the world with Meru at the center and to impose a scale and graticule on it. That these mapmakers represented the land in this way instead of using trigonometric measurements which would have been privileged in the Western tradition was apparently very much a choice: Pullè remarks that in the Middle Ages, trigonometry was used for sophisticated astronomical measurements, but not geographic ones in India, despite the fact that it was used for such purposes by the Arabs at that time (11–12).

6. It is often forgotten that the drawing that the uncouth Russians in Kipling's *Kim* think of as a piece of valuable native art, and try to steal from the Tibetan lama, is, among other things, a map. The Russians are there mapping the territory for a potential invasion, and of course, Kim is there to gain and destroy their data—he throws their cartographic instruments into a midden. Thus the contest for the land is played out cartographically.

7. For example, *Notes on the Medical Topography of Calcutta* by James Ranald Martin (1837) provided two maps, a detailed map of Calcutta in the mid-1700s and a topographic map of Bengal showing major waterways, and a fairly detailed overview of the growth of Calcutta as a British colonial city. Martin noted that the city's insalubrious location was typical of British colonial cities, as their founders were more concerned with having a good port and access to commercial transit than with the healthfulness of their sites (1). He goes on, however, to blame Calcutta's health problems equally on its moist geography and the natives' habits, as morally healthy inhabitants, he suggests, would have done something to drain the land.

8. I have, in the interest of manageability, not examined the vast body of meteorological charts which also accompany this literature. Although charts of windspeed, barometric pressure, and the like are simply maps of another kind, I have preferred to concentrate on those representations most visibly and directly connected to lived space. However, I would like to suggest that this literature progresses, becoming ever more subtle and sophisticated, attending to ozone levels (as Acland does for example) and tracing long-term repetitions of phenomena. From an early attention to prevailing winds and temperatures in specific localities, this literature increasingly comes to con-

nect to maps in its placement of communities, from areas in London to the British Isles more generally, in a larger world from which they cannot be separated and to which they are vulnerable, as they trace the movements of weather systems across maps of the world, for example. A peculiar instance of this using magnetism, rather than wind, is Lawson's cholerific wave map.

9. The map is engraved by T. Harwood, published by Burgess and Hill. Probably Orton traced or copied what he wanted from another map; perhaps he drew it.

10. He also refers to Moreau de Jonnes's work and, without mentioning the map, clearly refers to the argument of it.

11. There is no legend; the lines are explained on page xivi in a footnote: "The map has been engraved from a drawing prepared . . . by the Deputy Surveyor General: the engraving has not done justice to the drawing." An explanation of the red and yellow lines follows.

12. This map appears to have been constructed with different evidence (or, perhaps, standards of evidence) than Orton's. Although they cover the same period, and in most cases the dates coincide, Orton's maps show places as suffering from cholera that Scot does not (e.g., Darwar). (Scot is also not concerned with northern India, and so does not show, as Orton does, cholera extending about Nagpoor, where the lines of spread end abruptly instead of extending beyond the map.) Scot's map gives one the sense that the cholera went no further north directly over land than Asseerghun, whereas Orton clearly shows its extension as far north as Saharunpore. Obviously, Scot is concerned with the company's territories, whereas Orton is making a larger argument. Scot also does not show cholera's extension into Ceylon, the island below India that is partially visible on the map, whereas Orton shows the entire island. Orton can do this, in part, because his map of India is not topographically correct by later standards: distances are distorted, despite the general observance of the parallels, at least in regard to the placement of important cities. For example, in Orton's map, the southernmost tip of India, Cape Cormorin, is just below the eighth parallel, whereas in Scot's, the cape clears the top of the line with room to spare, and below the twentieth, Orton shows Jaulna substantially south of Aurungabad, whereas Scot places it only slightly south.

13. This map does have a legend:

Note: The course of the epidemic cholera in 1818–1819 is marked in Red lines along the principal roads. [Red is underlined in red] The crossroads and others mentioned in the narrative of progress are marked by Yellow lines [Yellow is underlined in Yellow]. [Then, larger, the title] Map shewing the principal places visited by the Epidemic Cholera in the Peninsula of India and the Dates of Its Commencement in 1818–1819.

14. An interesting early example of insular attitudes is James Kennedy, a London-based surgeon who appeared to have been "touring" during the epidemic, but who capitalized on the event by publishing a book in England on cholera in 1831. Having visited Bengal, but based in London and with the credibility that implies, Kennedy is able to make rather a good thing of his observations. Much of Kennedy's data appears to

have been taken from Scot, whom he acknowledges only equivocally. He uses the East India Company's data, and praises Scot rather ambiguously: "To record an opinion of the relative value of the Indian documents might seem an uncalled for, and invidious act, but I cannot omit stating, that the talents of Mr. Scot . . . claim peculiar respect. Mr. Scot executed a very difficult task with judgment and impartiality" (iv–v). Although he uses Scot's data, he draws up his own maps, probably having recourse to better documents in London than Scot was able to use: "Two Maps are given, illustrative of the geographical progress of cholera [here a footnote notes that Berlin and Vienna were added to the map but not the narrative before press]; and to render them the clearest and most correct, neither time nor attention has been spared" (vi). The maps show dates but not lines of spread, though sometimes two dates are shown to indicate a "repeated invasion" (vii).

The first long chapter, oddly, reads like a travelogue. Kennedy writes from the perspective of the naive traveller and assumes his reader is a Briton who has never been to India; after initially describing the picturesque beauties of India and the English settlement in Calcutta, he quickly gives way to criticism of the way one's "European tastes and habits are outraged" by India, emphasizing the constant disappointment of his expectations of exotic beauty. This he follows with the history of the epidemic. Far from emphasizing the similarity of Indian experience, the design of the narrative creates a sense of distance and difference from Britain, in which the whole discussion of the epidemic is framed.

Kennedy obviously intends the book to sell. It is 291 pages with only two small foldouts. The maps are carefully drawn by Kennedy himself, and engraved by R. Martin. The map of India differs from Orton's or Scot's, which show the coastal mountains, though it does show the two ranges bordering the north, toward Nepal. Like Orton, Kennedy includes the entire subcontinent and a portion of then-Afghanistan and Bengal. His map does not show as many places struck by cholera as Orton. Jubulpoor, for example, shows as clean of cholera on Kennedy, though he still displays the town itself. (This town is too far north to figure in Scot's map.) Kennedy's map shows no roads or lines of spread, though the argument is contagionist, as the title indicates. The second map shows "some of the principal places in Asia and Europe, visited by the Contagious Cholera from August 1817 to September 1834." The map is too small to be very detailed, including not only Asia and Europe but most of Africa and part of present-day Australia. It does not show the epidemics of most of western Europe that were to follow the volume's printing, and the data he has is quite incomplete. With the exception of Iceland in the top left corner, the map places the United Kingdom in the northwestern-most extreme of a larger world wherein cholera marches from India to the Far East and across the West. (In later maps, as more of Europe is required to be represented, India moves even further toward the border of the map, so that the overriding impression is of movement from east to west, as opposed to further east and south.)

India, however, is just right of center in Kennedy's map, and he emphasizes that the cholera did not only spread from east to west: "As contagious diseases, that can exist in different climates, have a disposition to extend in every direction, along the highways of human intercourse, we find that the cholera, even by sea, was not restricted to an Eastern route" but extended into China and the rest of Southeast Asia

(201). Kennedy also points out that the western spread began in a northern direction and then turned west. Still, these observations are framed within his comment in the beginning of the book: "The majority of the severe contagious diseases which have from time to time affected Europe, were imported from the East" (13), and he rather implies that India is intrinsically disease producing: "[W]e know that one species of tree will bear apples, another peaches. . . . The Malignant Cholera is indigenous in Bengal" (ix–x).

Kennedy's book went into a second edition in 1832. It is rarely cited by later medics; still, it is one of the few works based on observation of the cholera in India which had any circulation in the British Isles in the 1830s. In appealing to an insular audience, Kennedy used three tactics: legitimating himself as an insular practitioner, legitimating himself as an eyewitness while retaining the distance of a traveller, and placing India in a global context relevant to the Isles. In short, it is clear that he expected India to be interesting only as exotica and in its relation to domestic geography, not in its own right, and that his credibility is in direct proportion to his own identification with that domesticity.

CHAPTER 7. INDIA IN THE 1860s: MAPPING IMPERIAL DIFFERENCE

1. Even Kennedy, who emphasizes the strangeness of the landscape, rarely mentions the natives, and when he discusses them as patients, it is with the same attitude he would use for a European; in other words, if he others India, he is not concerned with doing so to the people, but the land. He does not blame or even refer to native habits, except in one instance, to refer to Muslim fasting as weakening the constitution, and does not implicate this in spreading the disease (223).

2. As Harrison discusses, European attitudes went from respect and interest in Indian beliefs and habits, including regarding medicine, in the early part of the century, to disregard and even contempt by the midcentury, a shift that parallels political changes in British relations to India.

3. Cornish is clearly not very interested in this report, and apparently detailed a native official to provide a map. The resulting document is quite large, covering all southern India at twelve miles to the inch; the unfolded map is approximately 6 ft. x 4.5 ft. Carefully and beautifully delineated, the "Map Illustrative of the Mortality from Cholera in the Madras Presidency during the Year 1869," drawn on transfer paper by V. Vardaraja Moodley of the Office of Sanitary Commissioner, is minimalist, showing major rivers and regional divisions, but no other detail. It, like the example mentioned above (Townsend), combines the general dot map (wherein dots mark places hit by cholera) with maps incorporating charts. It uses four colors, and each circle marks a place affected by cholera. The center of the circle may be divided in up to four parts, each filled by a different color: pink for European Troops, yellow for native troops, green for general population, and blue for prisoners. The rate of mortality, if known, is inscribed in each colored section. A circle surrounding the central circle is divided into twelve sections, each given a Roman numeral, representing

a month of the year. Another ring around this one follows the same divisions, and within each is the number of deaths for that month. Months with deaths are tinted brown. (These circular graphs probably owe something to the extensive use of similar graphs in the 1852 *Report on the Cholera Mortality of England in 1848–1849*). The report does not comment on this map much at all, except to say that it is not informationally complete and that it "has been prepared according to Dr. Goodeve's suggestions, but the Stational Diagrams make it very bulky. In future years a better form of map will be used" (1, footnote). The size of the round charts, which are also partially graphs (the portion related to month, for example), is related to the amount of data, not the population or mortality; the complexity of the data graphed precludes using simple visual correlations which would make data visible at a glance. It does, however, represent an aesthetically interesting and scientifically valid combination of chart and map properties. This type of technique is not much in evidence in insular maps after the 1852 report.

4. Lawson remarks that his map previously appeared in the 1864 *Statistical Reports on the Health of the Army*, but later he modified it in accordance with a map of Isoclinal magnetic lines in Johnson's *Physical Atlas*.

5. A good example of such a study (which rehistoricizes the land) is J. Forsyth's *Report on the Land Revenue Settlement of British Nimar: A District of the Central Provinces. 1868–1869*. This document gives a full historical background before and after British government, and relies in part on older Hindu land descriptions. It argues for improvement, in this case land irrigation, and in addition to a detailed analysis both historical and geological, it contains a map which shows "ancient and modern divisions" of the territory and includes "Old Pergunna" and "Old Tuppa" place-names. This is one of the emerging trend of studies in the late 1860s and 1870s, though by no means a dominant one yet, which begins to reinsert India into a historical tradition, and acknowledges that the land has changed over time and can be changed again.

6. The only example to the contrary I have found is the one drawn by Moodely, above, who uses what seems to be a fairly geographically accurate representation of the land in outline, though with few details, and pie graphs which operate as "spots," each representing a town hit by cholera, and each conveying complex information through numbers, colors, size, and so on, and the abstract map of spread from the Hurdwar fair. This is a map by a native, and Cornish felt the diagrams made the necessarily large map "too bulky" to reproduce in later reports.

AFTERWORD: STILL VISIBLE TODAY

1. The careful social engineering that structured localism in the USSR or the cluster in Singapore is often absent in efforts to localize in the West.

2. The maquiladora murders of Juarez in the late 1990s through the present bear witness to the special difficulties associated, in part, with the need for labor to travel considerable distances to the site of production.

3. Even Henri Lefebvre takes advantage of the cancer metaphor: "[T]he spread of urban tissue is accompanied by the fragmentation of the town. . . . [S]hould [the town] be sacrificed, letting the urban tissue proliferate in disorder and chaos but thereby strengthening the decision making centres?" (*The Survival of Capitalism* 28).

4. It should be said that I cannot do justice to Angotti and Hambleton's very nuanced arguments here, and am reducing their complexities rather crudely in the interests of an overall argument which I believe to be valid.

WORKS CITED

Abot, Samuel, trans. *Report to the International Sanitary Conference of a Commission from that Body on the Origin, Endemicity, Transmissibility and Propagation of Asiatic Cholera*. Boston: Mudge, 1867.

Acland, Henry Wentworth. "An Address to the Inhabitants of St. James's, Westminster on certain local circumstances affecting the health of rich and poor." London: Ridgway, 1847.

———. *Health. Address Delivered at the Social Science Congress at Plymouth*. Oxford and London: Parker, 1873.

———. "The Influence of Social and Sanitary Conditions on Religion: A Paper read by Desire at the Church Congress at Brighton, October 9, 1874." Oxford and London: Parker, 1874.

———. *Memoir on the Cholera at Oxford in the Year 1854, with Considerations Suggested by the Epidemic*. London: Churchill; Oxford: J. H. and J. Parker, 1856.

———. "Prints for Cottage Walls." London: Henry and Parker, 1862.

"An Address to the Inhabitants of St. James's, Westminster on Certain Local Circumstances Affecting the Health of Rich and Poor." London, James Ridgway, 1847.

"Analytical and Critical Reviews." *The British and Foreign Medical and Chirurgical Review*. January 1857. Reprinted as tract, no publication information.

Anderson, Benedict. *Imagined Communities: Reflections on the Origin and Spread of Nationalism*. London: Verso, 1983.

Angotti, Thomas. *Metropolis 2000: Planning, Poverty and Politics*. New York: Routledge, 1993.

Appendix. Report from Select Committees on East London Water Bills. Parliamentary Papers, Reports to Committees (original) Vol. 9, 1867.

Armstrong, Nancy. *Desire and Domestic Fiction. A Political History of the Novel*. Oxford: Oxford University Press, 1987.

Arnold, David. "Cholera and Colonialism in British India." *Past & Present* 113 (1986): 118–51.

————. *Colonizing the Body: State Medicine and Epidemic Disease in Nineteenth-Century India.* Berkeley: U of California P, 1993.

————, ed. *Imperial Medicine and Indigenous Societies.* Manchester: Manchester UP, 1988.

————. *The Problem of Nature: Environment, Culture, and European Expansion.* London: Blackwell, 1996.

————. "Social Crisis and Epidemic Disease in the Famines of Nineteenth-Century India." *Social History of Medicine* 6.3 (1993): 385–404.

Arnold, Matthew. *Culture and Anarchy.* (1882). Nov. 11, 2001. http://www.library. utoronto.ca/utel/nonfiction_u/arnoldm_ca/ca_ch1.html.

Arnott, Samuel. "An Address to the Inhabitants of St. Luke's, Berwick Street, particularly to those attending the church, on the late visitation of Cholera." London: Skeffington, 1854.

Aves, Ernest. "London as a Center of Trade and Industry." *Life and Labour of the People in London.* Ed. Charles Booth. Vol. 9. London: Macmillan, 1897. 176–88.

Baly, William, and William W. Gull. *Reports on Epidemic Cholera : Drawn up at the Desire of the Cholera Committee of the Royal College of Physicians.* London: Churchill, 1854.

Beames, Thomas. *The Rookeries of London: Past, Present, and Prospective.* 1850. 2nd Edition. London: Frank Cass, 1970.

Berghaus, Heinrich Carl Wilhelm. *Dr. H. Berghaus' Physikalischer Atlas, oder Sammlung von Karten, auf denen die hauptsachlichsten Erscheinungen der anorganischen und organischen Natur nach ihrer geographischen erbreitung und Vertheilung bildlich dargestellt sind.* 2 Bd. Gotha, 1845, 48.

Bewell, Alan. *Romanticism and Colonial Disease.* Baltimore: Johns Hopkins University Press, 1999.

Bickersteth, Edward. "God's Judgments in India a Warning to England." Preached at the Parish Church of St. Mary's, Aylesbury. London: Rivington, 1857.

Booth, Charles. *Charles Booth's London.* Ed. Fried and Elman. New York: Pantheon, 1968.

————, ed. *Life and Labour of the People in London.* 9 vols. London: Macmillan, 1897.

Brody, Howard, et al. "Map-Making and Myth-Making in Broad Street: The London Cholera Epidemic, 1854." *Lancet* 356. 9223 (July 1, 2000): 64–68.

Bryden, James L. *Cholera Epidemics of Recent Years viewed in relation to Former Epidemics, A Record of Cholera in the Bengal Presidency from 1817–1872.* Calcutta: Office of Supt. of Govt. Print., 1874.

————. *Epidemic Cholera in the Bengal Presidency: Report on the General Aspects of Epidemic Cholera in 1869: A Sequel to "A report on the cholera of 1866–68."* Calcutta: Office of Supt. of Govt. Print., 1870.

Buchanan, George. *St. Giles in 1857; being a report to the district board of works.* Sold at the Office of the Board of Works. June 4, 1858.

Buckland, William Dean. "A Sermon Preached in Westminster Abbey, on the 15th Day of November, 1849, being the Day of Thanksgiving to God for the Removal of the Cholera." London: John Murray, 1849.

Burford, Ephraim John. *Royal Saint James: Being a Story of Kings, Clubmen and Courtesans.* London: Hall, 1988.

Carroll, Lewis. *Sylvie and Bruno Concluded.* [1893] Dec. 1, 2002. http://ssl.serc.iisc.ernet.in/books/Fiction/Caroll/CompleteWorks/index.html.

Centers for Disease Control (CDC). "Overview of West Nile Virus 8/29/02." Dec. 11, 2002. www.cdc.gov/ncidod/dvbid/westnile/.

Chambers, W. F. *Three Lectures to Students at St. George's Hospital.* First lecture. *London Medical Gazette.* Feb. 9, 1849: 288–93.

"Cholera." *London Times.* Dec. 21, 1854: 7.

Christie, Alexander Turnbull. *A Treatise on the Epidemic Cholera.* London: Adland, 1833.

Clark, David. *Urban World/Global City.* London, Routledge, 1996.

Cooper, Charles Purton, Esq. "Letter to the Right Honorable Sir George Grey, B.T., M.P. [. . .] with Papers respecting the Sanitary State of part of the Parish of St. Giles in the Fields, London." 3rd ed. London: Pickering, 1850.

Corner, Miss. *The History of England from the Earliest Period to the Present Time Adapted to Youth, Schools and their Families.* London: Dean, 1870.

Cornish, William Robert. *Report on Cholera in Southern India for the Year 1869, with map illustrative of the disease.* Madras: Morgan, 1870.

Cowley, Geoffrey. "Breeding Grounds: As the AIDS Conference Opens in Spain, Scientists Are Finding New, Potentially Dangerous Viruses in the Monkeys of Central Africa." *Newsweek.* July 8, 2002: 48.

Crosby, Alfred W. *Ecological Imperialism: The Biological Expansion of Europe, 900–1900.* 1986. Cambridge: Cambridge UP, 1993.

Cuningham, James MacNab. *Report on the Cholera Epidemic of 1872 in Northern India.* Calcutta: Office of Supt. of Govt. Print., 1973.

David, Deirdre. *Fictions of Resolution in Three Victorian Novels.* New York: Columbia UP, 1981.

de Certeau, Michel. *The Practice of Everyday Life.* Trans. Steven F. Rendall. Berkeley: U of California P, 1984.

Delaporte, Francois. *Disease and Civilization: The Cholera in Paris, 1832.* Trans. Arthur Goldhammer; foreword by Paul Rabinow. Cambridge: MIT P, 1986.

Denton, J. Bailey. "Drainage of Lands and the Sewerage of Towns. A Paper on Model or Relief Mapping as the Best Index to the Capabilities of a Surface, with a description of the mode of constructing model maps." London: Weale, 1849.

Dickens, Charles. *Bleak House.* Oxford: Oxford UP, 1996.

———. *Letters of Charles Dickens.* Ed. Graham Storey et al. 11 vols. Oxford: Oxford UP, 1965.

———. *Martin Chuzzlewit.* Oxford: Oxford UP, 1989.

———. *Our Mutual Friend.* Oxford: Oxford UP, 1952.

———. *Sketches by Boz.* London: Chapman and Hall, 1900.

Dobie, Rowland. *History of the United Parishes of St. Giles in the Fields and St. George, Bloomsbury.* 2nd Ed. London: Henry Bickers, 1834. This copy is bundled with many other historical materials regarding the parish, generally not clearly sourced. In the collection of the British Library.

Donzelot, Jacques. *The Policing of Families.* Fwd. by Gilles Deleuze; trans. Robert Hurley. New York: Pantheon, 1979.

Douglas, Mary. *Purity and Danger : An Analysis of Concepts of Pollution and Taboo.* 1966. London : Routledge & Kegan Paul, 1980.

Durey, Michael. *The Return of the Plague: British Society and the Cholera, 1831–2.* Dublin : Gill and Macmillan, 1979.

Edney, Matthew H. *Mapping an Empire. The Geographical Construction of British India, 1765–1843.* 1990. Chicago: U of Chicago P, 1997.

Elliot, James. *The City in Maps: Urban Mapping to 1900.* London: British Library, 1987.

Elliott, Henry Venn. "Two Sermons on the Hundred and First and Sixty-Second Psalms as Applicable to the Harvest, the Cholera, and the War." London: Hatcherd, 1854.

Englander, David. "Booth's Jews: The Presentation of Jews and Judaism in Life and Labour of the People in London." *Retrieved Riches: Social Investigation in Britain 1914–1940.* Ed. David Englander and Rosemary O'Day. Ashgate, Eng.: Scolar, 1995. 289–322.

Evans, Richard J. *Death in Hamburg: Society and Politics in the Cholera Years, 1830–1910.* Oxford: Clarendon, 1987.

Farr, William. "Influence of Elevation on the Fatality of Cholera." *Journal of the Statistical Society of London* 15 (1852): 155–83.

———. *Report on the Cholera Epidemic of 1866 in England, supplement to the Twenty-Ninth Annual Report of the Registrar General.* London: Eyre and Spottiswoode, 1868.

———. *Report on the Mortality of Cholera in England: 1848–1849.* London: Clowes, 1852.

Faucher, Léon. "Extrait de la Revue des Deux Mondes, livraison du 1er novembre 1843. "Etudes sur L'Angleterre. No. II Saint-Giles." Paris: Fournier, 1843.

First Report of the Commissioners Appointed to Inquire into the Best Means of Preventing the Pollution of Rivers. (River Thames). 2 vols. London: Eyre and Spottiswoode, Her Majesty's Stationery Office, 1866.

Forbes, Anna. *Where Did AIDS Come From?* AIDS Awareness Library. New York: Rosen, 1996.

Forsyth, James. *Report on the Land Revenue Settlement of British Nimar: A District of the Central Provinces. 1868–1869.* Nagpore, India: Chief Commissioner's Office Press, 1870.

Foucault, Michel. *The Birth of the Clinic. An Archaeology of Medical Perception.* New York: Routledge, 1989.

———. "Governmentality." *The Foucault Effect: Studies in Governmentality.* Ed. Graham Burchell, Colin Gordon, and Peter Miller. Chicago: U of Chicago P, 1991.

Fraser, D., T. Hughes, and J. M. Ludlow. "Report on a Sanitary Inspection of the Golden Square District." Appendix. *Report of the Committee for Scientific Inquiries in relation to the Cholera Epidemic of 1854.* London: Eyre and Spottiswoode, 1855. 138–65.

Gallagher, Catherine. "The Bioeconomics of *Our Mutual Friend.*" *Subject to History.* Ithaca: Cornell UP, 1991.

Gardiner, Alfonzo. *How to Draw a Map.* London: Hughes, 1879.

Gavin, Hector. *Sanitary Ramblings. Being Sketches and Illustrations of Bethnal Green. A Type of the Condition of the Metropolis and other Large Towns.* London: Churchill, 1848.

General Board of Health. *Report of the General Board of Health on the Epidemic Cholera 1848 and 1849.* London: Clowes, 1850.

———. *Report on the Last Two Cholera Epidemics of London, as Affected by the Consumption of Impure Water.* London: Eyre and Spottiswoode, 1856.

General Board of Health Medical Council. Appendix. *Report of the Committee for Scientific Inquiries in Relation to the Cholera Epidemic of 1854.* London: Eyre and Spottiswoode, 1855.

Gilbert, E. W. "Pioneer Maps of Health and Disease in England." *Geographical Journal* 124 (1958): 172–83.

Gilbert, Pamela K. "Producing the Public: Public Medicine in Private Spaces." *Medicine, Health and the Public Sphere in Britain, 1600–2000.* London: Routledge, 2002. 43–59.

———. "'Scarcely To Be Described': Urban Extremes as Real Spaces and Mythic Places in the London Cholera Epidemic of 1854." *Nineteenth Century Studies* 14 (2000): 149–72.

———. "'A Sinful and Suffering Nation': Cholera and the Evolution of Medical and Religious Authority in Britain, 1832–1866." *Nineteenth Century Prose* 25.1 (Spring 1998): 35–59.

Glaisher, James. "Report upon the Meteorology of London, in relation to the Cholera Epidemic of 1853–4." Appendix 1. General Board of Health. *Report of the General Board of Health on the Epidemic Cholera 1848 and 1849.* London: Clowes, 1850. 1–118.

Glasheen, Joan. *St. James's, London.* Chichester, Eng.: Phillimore, 1987.

Godwin, George. *Town Swamps and Social Bridges.* London: Routledge, Warnes, and Routledge, 1859.

Gole, Susan. *Early Maps of India.* New York: Humanities Press, 1976.

Golledge, Reginald G., and Robert J. Stimson. *Spatial Behavior.* New York: Guilford, 1997.

Gould, Peter and Rodney White. *Mental Maps.* New York: Penguin, 1974.

Grainger, Richard Dugard. Appendix B. *Report of the General Board of Health on the Epidemic Cholera 1848 and 1849.* London: Clowes, 1850.

Hambleton, Robin. "Consumerism, Decentralisation and Local Democracy." *Managing the Metropolis. Metropolitan Renaissance: New Life for Old City Regions.* Ed. Peter Roberts et al. Avebury, Eng.: Aldershot, 1993.

Hamlin, Christopher. *Public Health and Social Justice in the Age of Chadwick: Britain, 1800–1854.* Cambridge: Cambridge UP, 1998.

Harley, John Brian. "Deconstructing the Map." *Cartographica* 26.2 (1989): 1–20.

Harrison, Mark. *Public Health in British India: Anglo-Indian Preventive Medicine, 1859–1914.* Cambridge: Cambridge UP, 1994.

Harvey, David. *Consciousness and the Urban Experience.* Baltimore: Johns Hopkins UP, 1985.

———. *The Urbanization of Capital.* Baltimore: Johns Hopkins UP, 1985.

Hassall, Arthur Hill. "Report on the Chemical Composition of Some London and Provincial Wells." Appendix. *Report of the Committee for Scientific Inquiries in Relation to the Cholera Epidemic of 1854.* London: Eyre and Spottiswoode, 1855. London: General Board of Health, Medical Council. 191–307.

Hawksley, Thomas, C. E. *Replies to the Queries issued by Her Majesty's Commissioners for inquiring into the present State of Large Towns &c., with additional observations in answer to the further inquiries of J. R. Martin.* London: Clowes, [n.d.].

Hewlett, Thomas Gillham. *Report of Measures Recommended in Bombay to Prevent Cholera Spreading Westward by the Sea towards European Nations.* Bombay: Education Society, 1867.

Howe, George Melvyn. "Medical Geography." *Geography Yesterday and Tomorrow.* Ed. E. H. Brown. Oxford: Oxford UP, 1980.

Hughes, T. Snead. "A Sermon Preached in the Parish Church of Corsham, Wiltshire Oct. 7, 1857 on the Day of Humiliation." London: Seeley, Jackson and Halliday, 1857.

Hughes, William. *A Manual of Mathematical Geography Comprehending an Inquiry into the Construction of Maps with Rules for the Formation of Map-projections.* 2nd ed. London: Longman, Brown, Green and Longmans, 1852.

India Office. *A Catalogue of Manuscript and Printed Reports, Field Books, Memoirs, Maps [. . .] of the Indian Surveys deposited in the Map Room of the India Office.* London: Allen, 1878.

Jackson, John. *Committee of Health and Sanitary Improvement. Report of the Proceedings of the Committee Upon the Inquiries Made by the Visitors as to the Sanitary Conditions of Certain Poor Districts of the Parish.* London: Brettell, 1848.

Jameson, James. *Report on the Epidemick Cholera Morbus, as it Visited the Territories subject to the Presidency of Bengal in the Years 1817, 1818, and 1819.* Calcutta: Balfour, 1820.

Jarcho, Saul. " The Contributions of Heinrich and Hermann Berghaus to Medical Cartography." *Journal of the History of Medicine and the Allied Sciences* 24 (1969): 412–15.

———. "Yellow Fever, Cholera, and the Beginnings of Medical Cartography." *Journal of the History of Medicine and the Allied Sciences* 25 (1970): 131–42.

Jarvis, Brian. *Postmodern Cartographies: The Geographical Imagination in Contemporary American Culture.* New York: St. Martin's, 1998.

Jerrold, Douglas. *The History of St. James and St. Giles.* Boston: Redding, 1847.

Kearns, Gerry, and Chris Philo. "Culture, History, Capital: A Critical Introduction to the Selling of Places." *Selling Spaces: The City as Cultural Capital, Past and Present.* Ed. Gerry Kearns and Chris Philo. New York: Pergamon, 1993.

Kearns, Robin A. "Place and Health: Towards a Reformed Medical Geography." *The Professional Geographer* 45 (1993): 139–47.

Keating, Peter J. *Into Unknown England, 1866–1913: Selections from the Social Explorers.* London: Fontana, 1976.

———. *The Working Classes in Victorian Fiction.* London: Routledge and Kegan Paul, 1971.

Kell, Edmund. "What Patriotism, Justice, and Christianity Demand for India: A Sermon preached Oct 11, 1857 at the Chapel, Canal Walk and Southampton" 4th ed. London: Whitfield, 1858.

Kennedy, James. *The History of the Contagious Cholera; with Facts Explanatory to its Origin and Laws, and of a Rational Method of Cure.* London: Cochrane, 1831.

King, Geoff. *Mapping Reality: An Exploration of Cultural Cartographies.* New York: St. Martin's, 1996.

Klein, Ira. "Cholera, Dysentery and Development in Eastern India 1871–1921." *Journal of Indian History: Golden Jubilee Volume* (1973): 805–20.

———. "Death in India, 1871–1921." *Journal of Asian Studies* 32.4 (1973): 639–59.

———. "Imperialism, Ecology and Disease: Cholera in India, 1850–1950." *Indian Economic and Social History Review* 31.4 (1994): 491–518.

Kotulak, Ronald. "AIDS Epidemic Shows No Letup In March Around the World." *Chicago Tribune* (December 22, 1985): 11. http://www.aegis.com/news/ct/1985/CT851207.html.

Kristeva, Julia. *Desire in Language: A Semiotic Approach to Literature and Art.* Trans. Thomas Gora, Alice Jardine, and Leon S. Roudiez. Ed. Leon S. Roudiez. New York: Columbia UP, 1980.

Kucich, John. *Excess and Restraint in the Novels of Charles Dickens.* Athens: U of Georgia P, 1981.

Kudlick, Catherine. *Cholera in Post-Revolutionary Paris: A Cultural History.* Berkeley: U of California P, 1996.

Lawson, Emily. *Through Tumult and Pestilence.* London: SPCK, 1886.

Lawson, Robert. "Further Observations on the Influence of Pandemic Waves in the Production of Fevers and Cholera." Paper presented March 2, 1868. *Transactions of the Epidemiological Society of London,* sessions 1866–1876. Vol. 3. 216–31.

Lea, John. *Cholera, with Reference to the Geological Theory.* Cincinnati: Wright, Ferris, 1850.

Leech Porter, J. "National Christianity for India, or National Acts and National Duties viewed in connection to the Sepoy Mutinies." London: Wertheim and Macintosh, 1857.

Lefebvre, Henri. *The Production of Space.* Trans. Donald Nicholson-Smith. Oxford: Blackwell, 1991.

———. *The Survival of Capitalism.* New York: St. Martin's, 1976.

Levi-Strauss, Claude. *Myth and Meaning.* London: Routledge and Kegan Paul, 1978.

———. *Structural Anthropology.* Trans. Claire Jacobson and Brooke Grundfest Schoepf. New York: Penguin, 1963.

London Cholera Hospital Casebooks. 1832. Manuscripts in the archive of the Royal College of Physicians.

Londres et Ses Environs. Paris: Chez Baily Frères, 1862.

Macpherson, John. *Cholera in its Home, with a Sketch of the Pathology and Treatment of the Disease.* London: Churchill, 1866.

Malleson, G. B. and Cunningham, J. M. *Report on the Cholera Epidemic of 1867 in Northern India.* Calcutta: Office of Supt. of Govt. Print., 1868.

Marcus, Sharon. *Apartment Stories: City and Home in Nineteenth-Century Paris and London.* Berkeley: U of California P, 1999.

Martin, James Ranald. *Notes on the Medical Topography of Calcutta.* Calcutta: Hutmann, 1837.

Massey, Doreen. *Space, Place and Gender.* Minneapolis: U of Minnesota P, 1994.

Maurice, Thomas. *Indian Antiquities* [. . .] . London: Printed for the author and sold by W. Richardson, 1794–1800.

Mayer, Jonathan D., and Melinda S. Meade. "A Reformed Medical Geography Reconsidered." *The Professional Geographer* 46 (1994): 103–06.

Mayhew, Henry. *London Labour and the London Poor*. New York: Penguin, 1985.

McClintock, Anne. *Imperial Leather: Race, Gender, and Sexuality in the Colonial Conquest*. New York: Routledge, 1995.

M'Cree, George Wilson. "Day and Night in St. Giles: A Lecture Delivered in the British Schoole Room, Bishop Auckland, on Tuesday June 17th, 1862." Rpt. from *Bishop Auckland Herald* June 21, 1862. No publication information.

Mehta, Uday Singh. *Liberalism and Empire: A Study in Nineteenth-Century British Liberal Thought*. Chicago: U of Chicago P, 1999.

"Metropolitan Confusions." *London City Press* (July 14, 1866): 4.

Metz, Nancy Aycock. "Discovering a World of Suffering: Fiction and the Rhetoric of Sanitary Reform, 1840–1860." *Nineteenth Century Contexts* 15.1 (1991): 65–81.

Michie, Helena. "'Who Is This in Pain?' Scarring, Disfigurement, and Female Identity in *Bleak House* and *Our Mutual Friend*." *Novel* 22.2 (1989): 199–212.

Miller, D. A. *The Novel and the Police*. Berkeley: U of California P, 1988.

Moretti, Franco. *Atlas of the European Novel, 1800–1900*. New York: Verso, 1998.

Morris, Robert John. *Cholera 1832: The Social Response to an Epidemic*. London: Croom Helm, 1976.

Nead, Lynda. *Victorian Babylon: People, Streets and Images in Nineteenth Century London*. New Haven: Yale UP, 2000.

Newton, Robert. Introduction. *The History of the Cholera in Exeter in 1832*. By Thomas Shapter. 1849. Wakefield and London: S. R. Republishers, 1971.

North Carolina Division of Environmental Health. "Public Health Pest management. West Nile Virus Alert." Nov. 2002. Dec. 19, 2002. http://www.deh.enr.state.nc.us/phpm/wnv/.

Oconee Pediatrics. "West Nile Virus." Dec. 11, 2002. www.oconeepediatrics.com/currenttopics.php.

O'Connor, Erin. *Raw Material: Producing Pathology in Victorian Culture*. Durham: Duke UP, 2000.

Ormerod, William Piers. *On The Sanatory Condition of Oxford*. Oxford: Ashmolean Society, 1848.

Orton, Reginald. *An Essay on the Epidemic Cholera of India*. 2nd ed., with a supplement. London: Burgess and Hill, 1831.

Osborne, Thomas, and Nikolas Rose. *Governing Cities: Liberalism, Neoliberalism and Advanced Liberalism*. Urban Studies Programme, Working Paper No. 19. Toronto: Urban Studies Programme, Division of Social Science, York U, April 1998.

Owen, Wilfred. "Mobility and the Metropolis." *Cities in a Global Society.* Ed. Richard V. Knight and Gary Gappert. Urban Affairs Annual Reviews 35. New York: Sage, 1989.

Parliamentary Papers. Session 1850. Vol. 21.

Pelling, Margaret. *Cholera, Fever and English Medicine, 1825–1865.* Oxford: Oxford UP, 1978.

Pike, David L. "Modernist Space and the Transformation of Underground London." *Imagined Londons.* Ed. Pamela K. Gilbert. Albany: State U of New York P, 2002. 101–20.

Poovey, Mary. *The History of the Modern Fact.* Chicago: U of Chicago P, 1998.

———. *Making a Social Body: British Cultural Formation, 1830–1864.* Chicago: U of Chicago P, 1995.

Prashad, Vijay. "Native Dirt/Imperial Ordure: The Cholera of 1832 and the Morbid Resolutions of Modernity." *Journal of Historical Sociology* 7.3 (1994): 243–60.

Pritchard, Allan. "The Urban Gothic of *Bleak House.*" *Nineteenth-Century Literature* 45.4 (Mar. 1991): 432–52.

Procacci, Giovanna. "Social Economy and the Government of Poverty." *The Foucault Effect: Studies in Governmentality.* Ed. Graham Burchell, Colin Gordon, and Peter Miller. Chicago: U of Chicago P, 1991. 151–68.

Pullè, Francesco Lorenzo. *La cartografia antica dell'India.* Firenze: Carnesecchi: 1901.

Ramasubban, Radhika. "Imperial Health in British India: 1857–1900." *Disease, Medicine and Empire.* Ed by Roy MacLeod and Milton Lewis. London: Routledge, 1988. 38–60.

Reeder, David. "Representations of Metropolis: Descriptions of the Social Environment in Life and Labour." *Retrieved Riches: Social Investigation in Britain 1914–1940.* Ed. David Englander and Rosemary O'Day. Ashgate: Scolar Press, 1995. 323–38.

Report of the Committee for Scientific Inquiries. Irish University Press Series of British Parliamentary Papers. Reports on the Epidemics of 1854 and 1866 and other Reports on Cholera with Appendices. Health, Infectious Diseases 3. Shannon, Ireland: Irish UP, 1970. 5–67.

Report of the General Board of Health on the Epidemic Cholera 1848 and 1849. London: Clowes, 1850.

Report on the Cholera Epidemic of 1866 in England, supplement to the Twenty-Ninth Annual Report of the Registrar General. London: Eyre and Spottiswoode, 1868.

Report on the Cholera Outbreak in the Parish of St. James's, Westminster, During the Autumn of 1854. Presented to the Vestry by the Cholera Inquiry Committee, July 1855. London: Churchill, 1855.

Report on the Mortality of Cholera in England: 1848–1849. London: Clowes, 1852.

Richards, Thomas. *The Imperial Archive: Knowledge and the Fantasy of Empire.* New York: Verso, 1993.

Richardson, Benjamin Ward. "John Snow M.D., A Representative of Medical Science and Art of the Victorian Era." *Snow on Cholera, Being a Reprint of Two Papers by John Snow M.D. With a Biographical Memoir by Benjamin Ward Richardson.* New York: Commonwealth Fund, 1936. xxiii–xlviii.

Rider, William. *Report to the General Board of Health on a Further Inquiry to the Boundaries [. . .] in the Parish of Haworth.* London: Eyre and Spottiswoode, [1853]. Bound in C. E. Hawksley Thomas, *Replies to the Queries issued by Her Majesty's Commissioners for inquiring into the present State of Large Towns &c., with additional observations in answer to the further inquiries of J. R. Martin.* London: W. Clowes and Sons, London, [n.d.].

Robinson, Arthur H. *Early Thematic Mapping in the History of Cartography.* Chicago: U of Chicago P, 1982.

———. "The 1834 Maps of Henry Drury Harness." *Geographical Journal* 121 (1955): 440–50.

Rose, Gillian. *Feminism and Geography: The Limits of Geographical Knowledge.* Minneapolis: U of Minnesota P, 1993.

Rose, Nikolas. *Powers of Freedom: Reframing Political Thought.* Cambridge: Cambridge UP, 1999.

Rosenberg, Charles E. *The Cholera Years: The United States in 1832, 1849, and 1866.* With a new afterword. Chicago: U of Chicago P, 1987.

Saint James, Westminster, Parish of. *Report on the Cholera Outbreak in the Parish of St. James, Westminster during the Autumn of 1854. Presented to the Vestry of the Cholera Inquiry Committee, July 1855.* London: Churchill, 1855.

Sanderson, William. "Suggestions in reference to The Present Cholera Epidemic, for the Purification of the Water Supply and the Reclamation of East London, with Remarks on the Origin of the Cholera Poison." London: Macintosh, 1866.

Schwarzbach, F. S. "*Bleak House:* The Social Pathology of Urban Life." *Literature and Medicine* 9 (1990): 93–104.

Scot, William. *Report on the Epidemic Cholera as it has appeared in the territories subject to The Presidency of Fort St. George.* Drawn up by order of government, under the superintendence of the medical board. Madras: Asylum P, 1824.

———. *Report on the Epidemic Cholera as it has appeared in the territories subject to The Presidency of Fort St. George.* Drawn up by order of government, under the superintendence of the medical board. Abridged from the original report printed at Madras in 1824, with introductory remarks, by the author. Edinburgh: Blackwood, 1849.

Shapter, Thomas. *The History of the Cholera in Exeter in 1832.* London: Churchill, 1849.

Simon, John. *Report on the Cholera Epidemic of 1854 as it Prevailed in the City of London.* London: Dawson, 1854.

——— . *Report on the Last Two Cholera Epidemics of London as Affected by the Consumption of Impure Water, addressed to the General Board of Health by the Medical Officer of the Board.* London: Eyre and Spottiswoode, 1856.

Sircar, D. C. *Studies in the Geography of Ancient and Medieval India.* Delhi: Motilal Banarsidass, 1971.

Smith, H. Llewelyn. "Influx of Population." *Life and Labour of the People in London.* Ed. Charles Booth. Vol.1. London: Macmillan, 1897. 501–63.

Smith, Neil. *Uneven Development : Nature, Capital, and the Production of Space.* New York: Blackwell, 1984.

Snow, John. Letter in *British Medical Journal* (1857): 864–65.

——— . Letter in *Edinburgh Medical Journal* 1 (1855–56): 668–70.

——— . *On the Mode of Communication of Cholera.* London: Churchill, 1849.

——— . *On the Mode of Communication of Cholera.* 2nd ed., enlarged. London: Churchill, 1855.

——— . "On the Pathology and Mode of Communication of Cholera." Rpt. from *London Medical Gazette* 44 (1849). No publication data.

——— . *Snow on Cholera, Being a Reprint of Two Papers by John Snow M.D. With a Biographical Memoir by Benjamin Ward Richardson.* New York: Commonwealth Fund, 1936.

Stallybrass, Peter, and Allon White. *The Politics and Poetics of Transgression.* Ithaca: Cornell UP, 1986.

Steig, Michael. "Dickens' Excremental Vision." *Victorian Studies* 8.3 (1970): 339–54.

Stevenson, Lloyd G. "Putting Disease on the Map: The Early Use of Spot Maps in the Study of Yellow Fever." *Journal of the History of Medicine and the Allied Sciences* 20 (1965): 226–61.

Stillwaggon, Eileen. "HIV/AIDS in Africa: Fertile Terrain." *Journal of Development Studies* 38.6.1 (August 2002): 22.

"Supplement to the Report of the Committee for Scientific Inquiries." *Irish University Press Series of British Parliamentary Papers. Reports on the Epidemics of 1854 and 1866 and other Reports on Cholera with Appendices. Health, Infectious Diseases 3.* Shannon, Ireland: Irish UP, 1970. 81–143.

Sussman, Herbert L. *Victorian Masculinities: Manhood and Masculine Poetics in Early Victorian Literature and Art.* Cambridge: Cambridge UP, 1995.

Sutherland, John, *Report on the Sanitary Condition of the Epidemic Districts in the United Parishes of St. Giles and St. George, Bloomsbury, with Special Reference to the Threatened Visitation of Epidemic Cholera.* London: Eyre and Spottiswoode, 1852.

Taylor, Gordon. "Saint Giles in the Fields: Its Part in History" 1971, 4th ed. N.p., 1980.

Thai-Ker, Liu. "From Megacity to Constellation City: Towards Sustainable Asian Cities." *Megacities, Labour and Comunications.* Ed. by Toh Thian Ser. Singapore: Institute of Southeast Asian Studies, 1998. 3–26.

Thomson, R. D. "Report on the Examination of Certain Atmospheres during the Epidemic of Cholera." Appendix. General Board of Health, Medical Council. London: Eyre and Spottiswoode, 1855. 119–33.

Thompson, W. A. "Report on an Epidemic of Cholera at Thayetmoo, British Burmah, in 1869, especially with reference to its appearance in the Right Wing of Her Majesty's 76th Regiment." Cornish 46–79.

Thrower, Norman J. W. *Maps and Civilization: Cartography in Culture and Society.* Chicago: U of Chicago P, 1996.

——— . *Maps and Man: An Examination of Cartography in Relation to Culture and Civilization.* Upper Saddle River: Prentice Hall, 1972.

Townsend, S. C. *Report on the Cholera Epidemic of 1868.* N.p.: n.p., 1869. Bound with Malleson and Cuningham.

Tyner, Judith. "Geography Through the Needle's Eye." *The Map Collector* 66 (1994): 2–7.

United States Senate. 106th Congress, 2nd Session. *United Nations' Policy in Africa: Hearing Before the Committee on Foreign Relations.* S. Hrg. 106–872. July 12, 2000. From the U.S. Government Printing Office via GPO Access (DOCID: f:67707.wais) Oct. 3, 2002. http://frwebgate.access.gpo.gov/cgi-bin/getdoc.cgi?dbname=106_senate_hearings&docid=f:67707.wais.

Upton , Dr. *Dáil Éireann: Díospóireachtaí Parlaiminte (Irish Parliamentary Debates).* 434 (Oct. 6, 1993). Dec. 9, 2002. www.oireachtas-debates.gov.ie/D/ 0434/D. 0434.199310060308.html.

A Week in London; or, how to view the metropolis, with all its national establishments, Public Buildings, Exhibitions, Etc, in seven days, to which is prefixed a historical and descriptive Account of the Great City, from the Earliest Period to the Present Time. A New Edition. 6th ed. revised and enlarged. London: Craddock and Co., 1842.

WHO. *Basic Documents.* WHO. 16th ed. 1965.

Whitehead, Henry. *The Cholera in Berwick Street.* By the Curate of St. Luke's. 2nd ed. London: Hope, 1854.

Whittaker, D. K. "The Cholera Conference." *London Quarterly Review* 27 (Jan. 1867): 16–29.

Wilford, Francis. "An Essay on the Sacred Isles of the West, with Other Essays connected with that Work," *Asiatic Researches* X, 1808: 264–306.

Wolfreys, Julian. *Writing London: The Trace of the Urban Text from Blake to Dickens.* Basingstoke, Eng.: Macmillan; New York: St. Martin's, 1998.

Wood, Denis. *The Power of Maps.* New York: Guilford, 1992.

Wright, Kay Hetherly. "The Grotesque and Urban Chaos in *Bleak House.*" *Dickens Studies Annual: Essays on Victorian Fiction* 21 (1992): 97–112.

York, Mr. "Mr. York's Report." *Report on the Cholera Outbreak in the Parish of St. James's, Westminster, During the Autumn of 1854.* London: Churchill, 1855. 170–74.

INDEX